Being Healthy Can Kill You

Reading This Book Could Save Your Life

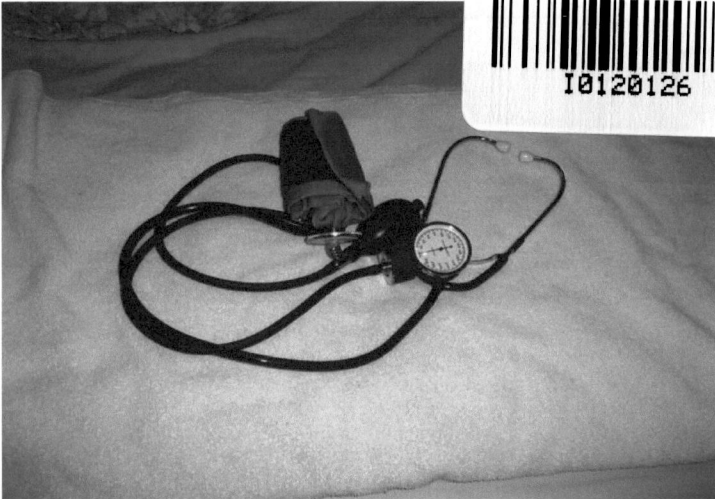

By Helen C. Ayers

Second Edition

Other Books by this Author

Appalachian Daughter, April, 2006
The Stuff of Legends, November, 2006
MURDER, Relatively Speaking, March 2010
Grandma's Brown County Cookbook, October, 2015
Devil's Halo, February, 2021
Granny Goes to the Cruise Ship (Granny Goosefoot Adventures Book 1), May, 2021
Granny Goosefoot Goes to New York (Granny Goosefoot Adventures), December, 2022
Harriet Goes to Dinner, August, 2022
The Frog and the Toad, February, 2023
The Bird Who Could Not Sing, July 2023
This Is Our Brown County Then 1800-1900: Revering Our Past, August, 2023

My favorite critics, (my readers) said this about my books:

"Her books are hilarious, truthful, sometimes sad, and should be made into a movie," many have said this.

"I laughed and I cried all the way through."

"This is the first book I ever read from one cover to the other and enjoyed every word and page."

"I stayed up all night reading her books. I could not put them down."

"This is a very talented and gifted author."

"I sincerely hope she writes many more down-home type books.

One doctor who entered my hospital room last summer had this to say about this particular book.

"This is the best book about health care I have ever read or heard about. It was precisely written by someone who knew the correct terminology. It is a marvel of perfection. This book should be a must read for every health care worker in the profession."

Then he walked out the door.

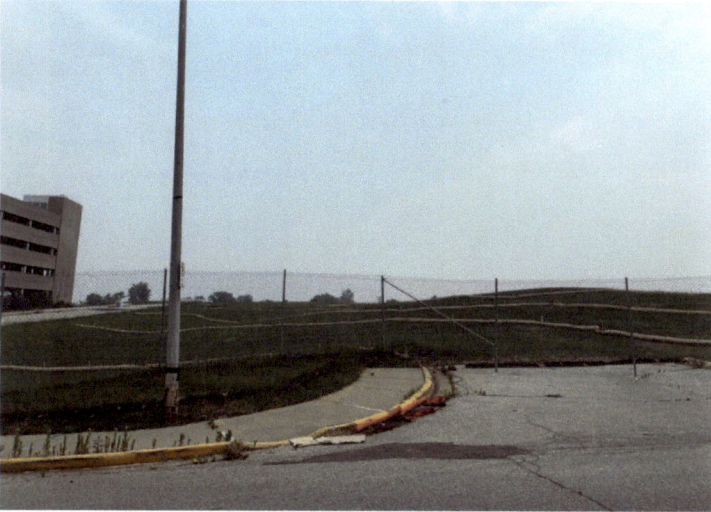

I would like to thank all the wonderful people in the health care industry who go that extra mile to make sure that the care they provide their patients is of the highest quality. I thank my husband for being my health care advocate through so many life threatening trials in the past few years. I would also like to thank my two sons for the love and support they give me. And especially I would like to thank my readers and friends who keep encouraging me to keep writing.

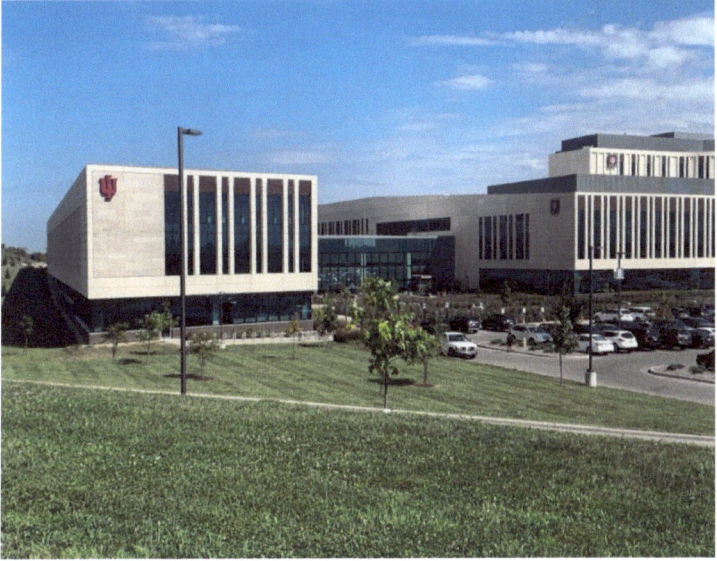

Being Healthy
Can Kill You

Reading This Book Could Save Your Life

Table of Contents

Today's Health Care

Modern medicine is a totally amazing and wonderful thing. It has become almost commonplace that if you need a new heart, liver, kidney, eye or various other body parts, you may have one simply by your doctor placing your name on a national or regional waiting list for spare parts. When a donated organ becomes available, matches your DNA as closely as possible, and your name is at the top of the list, the part becomes yours.

Those spare parts may come from either living donors, (most usually a close relative), or from a cadaver (dead person). A living donor can give a loved one or matching stranger a kidney or a piece of their liver and not suffer too many consequences. Giving this generous gift may allow someone to live a near normal life span. Obviously those spare parts from cadavers would include other transplantable organs that a living person needs himself to survive and which only become available upon one's death.

Either way you look at it, parts are parts, and if you are sick enough you will be glad to get an organ from any source. And, no it is not true that if you receive one of these spare parts from a cadaver that you will suddenly take on the characteristics of that dead person. Contrary to popular book and movie topics, this just does not happen.

This sharing of replacement body parts is the truly most outstanding advances in the modern world of medical care. Thousands of people have been made well, or nearly so, in this manner. The recipient usually has to take anti-rejection drugs for the rest of their life but they will be able to continue life in a pretty good manner. Taking these necessary medicines is a small price to pay for good health.

Even more remarkable are the advances in stem cell research. Scientists are attempting to develop a way by which if you need a new heart, for instance, they can take some of your own heart DNA and actually grow one for you. Once that new substance is injected back within your own heart it will then heal itself and no anti-rejection drugs will be necessary.

Not really, of course, I realize this statement is greatly over-simplified—but the upshot is, that is exactly what they are attempting to do. The initial growth of the DNA in a laboratory petri dish might just be a few stem cells but those cells can be injected into your own heart muscle or kidney, etc. and it is generally believed today that your body will, in time, cure itself. Only time will tell if this advance is successful.

This medical advance is just underway at this writing, but one day this Star Wars type medicine could become a reality. Researchers are close to that point right now if you can believe the stories in the daily newspapers, but many ethical questions remain.

Those of us who are familiar with the old Star Trek television series have seen a doctor wave a wand of some type along the entire body to diagnose what ailed a member of the ship's crew. That is coming closer and closer to today's medical advances. It is much closer than one might think.

I firmly believe that one day there will be no need for prisons unless it is just for corporal punishment of criminals.

Research continues in many areas regarding the brain cells of humans. Scientists are finding out new things every day about how the brain operates and utilizes the information it receives.

Sometime in the not-too-distant future they may develop a means of inserting a probe into the brain of a criminal and freezing or stunning a cell or two that will make it impossible for him to ever again commit the crime for which he stands accused. As scientists learn more and more about the human brain and how it works, they will be able to pinpoint the exact spot in that gray matter we all carry around in our skulls that make us do what we do.

If we commit a murder or rape someone, for instance, they can pinpoint and freeze that portion of our brain permanently to obliterate those urges. There will be no need for capital punishment because that person physically cannot commit that same crime again nor even have the urge to do so. He may commit other crimes, but his brain will be functionally unable to tell him, and he will have no inclination, to do the original crime again.

Won't it be a happy day in the morning when we do not have to kill a fellow human being for killing another human being and have that criminal's death on our own conscience? It will not bring back the person that has been murdered, but it will take away our own guilt of having to kill someone else to atone for what a criminal has done.

I think the trade off will be worth it. The freezing or deadening of that portion of the brain which made him commit a crime will not have any effect on the remainder of the person's brain cells. He will be able to function normally in society in all other respects but he just will not be able to commit the same type of crime ever again. Star Wars medicine? You betcha it is but we are getting there.

Some of these modern advances in medicine are just now on the horizon. The heart transplant procedures have been around since the mid 1960's. Kidney dialysis—mechanically cleansing the blood with a machine after your own kidneys have stopped working—and replacement of corneas has been a common practice for decades. Now surgeons are replacing almost a person's insides in one operation. They can replace the entire heart and lungs in quick order, or the whole intestinal system at one whack. Many other foreseen and unforeseen advances may not be here in my lifetime, but they may in yours.

A History Lesson

Most of us like to believe that our health care provider will take care of us from the cradle to the grave and do a good job all along the way. In many cases, this is true—but sadly, in others it is not. This has been true from ancient times to the present day. In ancient times, the doctor sometimes helped you into an early grave. In other words, like a skilled carpenter who can cover his mistakes, the doctor "buried his mistakes," and most of our relatives were none the wiser. Some doctors, unfortunately, still do so today.

The old time doctor, who might have also been your barber, (they often served both needs) may have been your worst enemy with his sometimes questionable cures and incompetent treatments.

I remember as a child being taken to the local sawbones when I was ill. This man, who was probably 85 or 90 years old at that time, would go into his dark and musty backroom and dig around in several jars, selecting and counting out pills. As he worked one could hear the clink and rattle of the pills against the glass jar as he ran his bare hand around inside that jar selecting your medications.

He would not have had many to choose from in those days and he never wrote a prescription but sold the drugs out of his own office rather than send you to a drugstore. The doctor would place the pills he had chosen for you, and now held in his bare hand, into a small white envelope on which he would have already written his instructions for taking the medicine.

The doctor **licked** the envelope's flap and sealed it down, leaving one corner of the envelope sticking up which he would then tuck inside to form the seal for the package. When this triangular flap was re-opened, a pouring spout was thus created for removing the pills. Just think, with the DNA technology we have today, how many doctor's identities could be determined from these little flaps.

I remember being about two or three years old and living in the mountains of Eastern Kentucky. A doctor had given my mother some very powerful pain pills in this type of dispenser. Like most toddlers and being curious as a cat, I had watched as Mother placed this package high up in a kitchen cupboard and I had bided my time.

One day when she and other adult relatives were busily wallpapering the dining room and ignoring the children at their feet, I climbed up onto the cabinet's pullout shelf and found those pills.

This was the type of cabinet which stood alone, had a flour sifter, built-in cutting board, and several doors, drawers and a pull-down door all of which is now known as a "Hoosier Cabinet."

There was a pull-out work table in the very middle of this cabinet which made it very easy for me as a small child to climb upon it. I did this by pulling out the lower drawers and using them as steps to this work table that I could then stand upon to explore the contents of this fascinating cabinet.

I, being far too young at that time to know any better, and probably thinking the pills were candy or something, poured those pills into my mouth and began chewing them.

Luckily for me Mother happened to see me standing on the cabinet busily chewing something and holding that white paper package in my hand. She immediately comprehended the danger I was in. She grabbed me up into her arms and forced my mouth open, swept my mouth with her finger and rushed me to the doctor whose office was perhaps ten miles distant. By the time we arrived at the doctor's office I was unconscious.

I was forcibly given an emetic, probably ipecac because it was very vile tasting and bitter, to make me throw up any of the pills that I might have swallowed. They determined I had not yet swallowed any of them but I had already absorbed so much of that medicine through my saliva that I went into a deep sleep.

When I woke many hours (it could have been days) later they found I could no longer walk or talk and I was very dizzy. I had to relearn my motor and speech skills all over again. I can vaguely remember this incident.

For this reason, I am very glad today that all medications are placed in childproof containers. If you have no young children who live in or visit your household and you have trouble opening these child-proof containers you may still ask your pharmacist to place your medicines in push-off top containers.

At other times when you were visiting an old-time doctor you might see him pulling out various bottles and containers in that dingy back room, removing a tad of this and a pinch or two of that and placing it in a mortar and pestle device.

After a lot of what appeared to be nearly magical hocus pocus, this powdered concoction might have been tapped out onto a small square of white paper, then rolled up and twisted at each end. The doctor would explain to us how to take this medicine for whatever had ailed us. Sometimes it worked, sometimes it didn't, but that never stopped him from practicing his apothecary talents on us.

This mortar and pestle device was rarely if ever cleaned thoroughly between uses. When accepting medicines formulated this way you might be given many different bits of the various other medicines prepared in it previously, the residue of which remained in that bowl. The doctor might occasionally turn the device over and thump it against his leg or blow hard down into it to remove drug residue or dust, but it was rarely thoroughly cleaned or sterilized.

If all else failed our parents would have been advised to physic us. This was accomplished by giving us a big dose of castor oil. It was believed that if your bowels moved regularly that all the germs in your body would be expelled naturally and castor oil helped things along splendidly. What I find castor oil useful for today is to take a small amount of it and rub it on my arthritic knees and fingers to relieve the pain. (Yes, it does work great!)

For confirmation of what I am saying here about old time medical care, leaf through any ancient medical book or document. The doctors were portrayed wearing bloody aprons, their bare hands deep down inside a screaming man's body as they forcibly removed some organ or another. The doctor usually had two or three burly assistants helping to hold his patient in place. They had few means of tranquilizing a patient other than offering as much whiskey or other spirits to drink as it took to make the patient pass out, so the patient often woke up from his inebriated stupor when the pain became too excruciating to bear. The doctor sometimes did not realistically expect his patient to survive his ministrations, nor perhaps actually cared whether he did or not. He was practicing medicine and this was all they knew at that time.

At one time blood letting was widely believed by doctors to cure almost any disease. Most of the time anymore, now that we are smarter and more modern, we know it is the act of replacing more blood inside the body's veins than is bleeding out that saves lives. Yet for hundreds of years barbers and doctors practiced this barbaric, useless and often fatal treatment.

A barber's or a doctor's assistants would hold down the patient's head, arms and feet while the doctor made a slit into an artery or one of the veins in a patient's elbows. A sufficient amount of blood would be released that the disease or infection was believed to have been drained from the patient's body or the patient eventually died.

Since this cure might be practiced day after day for several days and the patient lost so much strength they could no longer survive, they died due to blood loss. It was the lucky person in those days whose family did not call for the doctor's assistance. These practices served their purposes though because as doctors learned what was inside a living body and how the living body worked, they learned how to cure many of the problems of mortal humans, thus bringing us forward almost into the modern age of medical technology.

During the Civil War and even up through the early 1900s, if a soldier had been wounded in the leg or arm, infection set in almost before his body hit the ground. When that happened, gangrene often occurred and it was deadly. When gangrene hits your kidneys you were a dead duck, a local doctor friend explained to me one time when I was very, very ill.

Since that was before the advent of modern antibiotics, amputation became the normal way of saving the soldier's lives. Doctors in field tent hospitals wearing their white coats or rubber aprons covered with blood would have piles of arms and legs lying outside the operating tent theater at days end.

At that time in medical history whiskey, chloroform or laudanum might be the only anesthetic or pain control available to the doctor. Sometimes even those were unavailable and the soldier would be forcibly held down by others so his infected limb could be sawn off.

If the soldier survived this treatment, followed by a brief healing time, he would be allowed to go home. It was generally up to him how he got home. He might be provided with a crutch made from a forked limb, but sometimes he fended for himself as best he could.

By the time the Second World War occurred however, penicillin had been discovered and this one medicine alone served to save the lives of countless thousands of soldiers and moved us one step closer to modern medicine.

Also by that time, aspirin and morphine was in wide general use and ether was the preferred anesthetic; hand washing with soap and lots of water was encouraged for all medical personnel and various other means of personal hygiene by doctors was becoming commonplace.

Times were a-changing for sure.

Moving Forward

Today there are many capable health care professionals who are out there practicing their craft in whatever specialty happens to be theirs. They are there because they truly believe in the Hippocratic Oath they swore to uphold when they became licensed doctors. Sometimes their cures are truly miraculous. They have come a long, long way forward in the practice of medicine but there is still a long way to go also.

A very, very rare small number (thankfully) of medical professionals are out there practicing medicine for no other reason than because of the money they can earn. Liking their job and doing it well has nothing at all to do with engaging in their chosen profession.

Perhaps they were pressured by their families to become involved in the health care industry and they never got the nerve to go against that family pressure. But for whatever reason, these are the ones to be watchful of.

Your onus is in recognizing them; your reward is surviving their treatment if you don't recognize them.

Changing Doctors

For a variety of reasons unrelated to their skills, we sometimes must change our primary care physician.

For instance, when you change jobs you may be involved with a different HMO, or the company paid insurance plan where you now work changes. It now requires that you see only those physicians on a preferred provider list which they give you. You may be told to change primary care providers or lose health care coverage.

Other times you may find you have discovered you questioned the recommended course of treatment with your regular doctor that you have been seeing for many years and you now wish to see someone new.

For whatever reason, and there are a variety of reasons—a change of one's primary care physician (PCP) becomes necessary—and you must find a new one. Let the hunt begin.

Please, if this happens to you, spend some time talking to your friends and family, asking them which doctor they see. Ask if they are happy with their provider. Would they give him/her a great recommendation?

You may also call the local medical association for their recommendation and find out which one might be accepting new patients. Ask if they know of any complaints lodged against a particular doctor by his patients that you are considering seeing. Sometimes they will answer this last question and sometimes they will not respond. They might, either knowingly or unknowingly, even help to cover some doctor's mistakes.

Look for the local medical association's number in the yellow pages of your phone book, or call your county health department or a local hospital. Is there one particular doctor that perhaps specializes in a chronic condition you now have? If there is one, you might be wise to investigate this one further.

Finally, pay for a private consultation with the one you are thinking of choosing. Ask questions such as; "I have Crohn's disease (or any other chronic problem you may have), what would you recommend as a course of treatment. Can you treat that and what treatment method would you prefer and recommend?" Ask if he refers his patients to a specialist for some types of problems. Know ahead of time the answers you should expect to receive about the questions you will be asking this doctor. A little research will reveal the accepted normal methods of treatment for most diseases. The Internet and your public library are rife with medical knowledge. There is no excuse for medical ignorance, no matter how much or how little education you may have yourself, in this day and age. You can always ask someone you know and trust and whom you believe is more

knowledgeable than you, for their opinion.

Ask if he/she performs surgeries or would you be referred to another doctor who specializes in surgery should you need to have it. If referrals are the norm, then ask if the referred surgeon has the knowledge and skills for your particular medical problem. For instance, why should you see a general surgeon when you need brain or thoracic (chest) surgery? Practice makes perfect as the old saying goes, so you want the one surgeon with the absolute most successful percentage of surgeries in your particular area of need. Equally important is to also find out what his failure rate might be.

Ask which hospital your doctor is affiliated with. If his answer is none, walk away.

You want a health care provider who is recognized in his field and who is on staff of at least one or more hospitals in the area.

You may also elect to turn down a particular doctor because he is not affiliated with a hospital you have previously been a patient at and are satisfied with its level of care. This can be one of the most important questions you ask during the initial interview.

Also tell the doctor you are interviewing that you will be taking an active part in decisions concerning your health care. Explain to him that you don't want him to hurry you through examinations; you want things explained, in writing if necessary, for you to understand his instructions. If it takes half an hour you don't want them to object and you do not want to be rushed. This is vital to your survival.

If the doctor does object, or acts rushed, keep looking, because this doctor is not for you.

A good doctor should welcome the interest you show in your own health care and he should provide you with answers to your questions.

But be fair with him/her. Write down all your questions and complaints ahead of time so his time is not wasted while you fumble for words and so you won't forget to ask important questions.

You should make the decision to see this doctor as a patient on a regular basis and submit to being physically examined only when you are totally satisfied with the answers you have been given during this initial interview.

Even after all this initial contact, you must still take nothing for granted.

Doctors see many patients each day so it may be difficult for him to keep focused about your problems, but you see only one patient, yourself. Keep that in mind.

You can and may die if you or your doctor make the wrong decision regarding your health care.

The Nitty Gritty

Once upon a time I trusted almost all my doctors to make the best, most informed decisions about my health care. I had made my complaints to them and they had asked me a few questions. Perhaps they had run a few tests or taken some x-rays or scans to confirm their and my suspicions.

They were the ones who were educated, not I—they should have known more about my body than I did. Now I know better and I do not totally trust any of them no matter how many dusty diplomas they may have hanging askew on the walls of their office.

After you have nearly died a couple of times or more as I and my husband have done because of our doctor's inappropriate actions or simply plain incompetence, you learn that you know some things about your body that they do not know.

Oh, sure, they can run tests and find out many things that you cannot do for yourself, but only you know where it hurts, how badly it hurts, when it started hurting, etc. It is sometimes difficult to accurately describe pain and too, since pain and fever are not diseases but rather are indicators of diseases, you should also know that both fever and pain often mask the real underlying problem.

Sometimes your doctor won't particularly care that you are hurting and say "you're tough, take two ibuprofen (or aspirin) for pain every four hours, and if you aren't better in a couple of days, come back in to see me," then he will rush out of your exam room to see his next patient.

After all, seeing patients is how he makes a living, not only for himself but for the other members of his office staff who depend upon him for a paycheck. The more patients he sees during a normal workday, the better he can meet his expenses. If he has six or so exam rooms, the nurses will see that all are full throughout the day. If he has six rooms, then six patients will most likely share the same appointment time slot as you. The nurses will do the initial workups for your visit and record your answers so the doctor does not have to do the very routine exams and can drift from room to room as necessary.

But in his quest to earn a living he may neglect to look for the underlying cause of your pain altogether. Sometimes instead of ibuprofen or aspirin you might need Demerol, codeine, morphine, an antibiotic or some hardier medication to cure your problems.

Tell the doctor how badly you are hurting. Your pain is something he cannot detect or feel on his own but there is no excuse for him/her neglecting to look for the underlying cause of your pain.

This reminds me of an e-mail I recently received. I'm sorry ladies, but it is a blonde joke. **"A woman went to her doctor and said she hurt terribly all over her body, wherever she was touched.** He did not believe her and told her to demonstrate. **Using her right index finger, she pushed on her left shoulder and hollered loudly. She did the same to her belly and then to her knee, yelling after each place she touched.** He said to her, **"Stop, I have seen enough, it is your finger that is broken."**

He had found her underlying cause of pain.

I now question everything doctors tell me, and I ask for explanations both before and after any test is run.

Before the test I might ask, "Why are you running this test? What do you expect to find? Maybe even, how much will it cost me?" Keep a diary of each illness and his responses. Sometimes these tests are not really necessary or you realize you cannot afford to have them run. It that is the case, tell him right upfront that you cannot pay for them. Often other, less expensive tests can reveal what is wrong with you.

After the test results are known, I ask him to explain the results he obtained and you should too. Update your personal diary at this point and every step along the way.

Was the result of the test what your doctor had originally told you it probably would show? If it was not, ask him to explain the difference.

I now also ask for printed copies of the procedures and test results for my personal health-care file that I keep at home.

I want to know what my blood pressure reading is—is it high or low; what my blood sugar numbers are; and what my cholesterol numbers mean. Can I improve these numbers with diet and exercise alone or do I need medication or supplements to help me control these problems. How can I improve these figures without taking prescription medications? Will alternative herb remedies or acupuncture do the same thing without all the aggravating and sometimes life-threatening side effects of prescription drugs?

How many times have you gone to a doctor with one complaint and been given medicine for that only to discover that you now have a new complaint as a result of taking that medicine? Many times I am sure.

It is so easy to fall into the drug taking practice chosen by many doctors. But for every medicine you put into your body, there could be an adverse reaction. Some patients are more susceptible than others. Sometimes, too, drugs are a cop-out. You may be given something to allay your fears—these drugs are known as placebos—and your complaint can be ignored by your doctor.

The elderly are a very susceptible class of patient. Their aging bodies are sometimes nearly worn out. They fall victim to ailment after ailment. Often they are over-medicated to the extreme that they die. Why?

It is very simple. Many drug companies push their new and miraculous (according to them) drugs into the hands of the doctors who, in turn, generously add them to the daily drug cocktails of the elderly.

The elderly are the only class of people I know of who see their doctors on a regular recurring schedule.

The elderly not only have yearly physicals, they are repeat customers again and again throughout each year. Despite what many doctors claim about not wanting to take Medicare patients, they are a steady source of income to him.

Doctors give these elderly people a new drug and say, "I want to see you again in two weeks or two months." And those same people are right back in his office when the scheduled appointment appears on their calendars.

These same doctors will refer many of these elderly patients to first one specialist then another thus spreading the wealth even more. Those specialists they are referred to might give them another medicine or two or three to add to their daily cocktail of medicines.

This is how our elderly population can so easily become over-medicated.

The more you medicate some of these elderly patients, the worse their symptoms become until finally some simply die. They die not as a result of their ailments necessarily, but because of the high-powered medicines they have been advised by their doctors to consume. Many are afraid to refuse or even question the need to take the medicines their doctors prescribe.

The elderly class of people living today still contains a large number of poorly educated individuals. I am not saying they are stupid or dumb by any means, but they grew into adulthood when compulsory education did not exist. They are easily scared into taking these medications and would never think to question their doctor. The most literate of this group might sit up and question the necessity of taking the drugs.

It is hoped that all those reading this small book will sit up and take notice.

The life span of today's senior population is growing by leaps and bounds. They retire at a far younger age than their ancestors did and they live far longer than they did. Baby boomers are now reaching retirement age and this insured senior group of educated elderly will nearly burst the seams of a lot of doctor's offices and the doctors will love them. Guaranteed.

Younger people and children usually go to doctors only when they are actually sick, need inoculations or sports physical. They may or may not be covered by insurance plans so their visits are more sporadic and less profitable. Not so with the elderly. We are covered with Medicare!

How many children do you know who do not have dental coverage for such things through their parent's workplace, yet have braces on their teeth, for instance? Few, if any do, because the parents cannot personally afford to have it done. Their children survive and live a wonderful life with perhaps a tooth slightly gapped or a bit askew. The same thing is true in all areas of health care. Only those with an insurance card or cash in their hands are able to get into most doctor's offices.

That one little card—maybe two if you also have Medicare and a supplement or Medicaid—is the first thing the receptionist will ask you to produce when you see a new doctor for the first time.

Your insurance cards are the most important things in your wallet.

Medication

I want to know what each medication prescribed for me is to be used for and I want that information printed on every medicine bottle's label. At my age I sometimes forget why the medicine was prescribed, especially if it has some fancy name or I don't have to use it every day or if I am taking several medications on a daily basis. You simply forget, so the label should briefly describe what it is to be used for.

For instance, the printed label should say something very simple like, "Take one pill by mouth every four hours as needed for pain, or for blood pressure, etc." There is an old joke about taking medicine by mouth or as a suppository for hemorrhoids. I will not get into that one now but grandma used to tell it to me and laugh hysterically.

Instructions should be written in the commonly accepted language the ordinary patient can read and understand. If you speak a language other than English, then ask that the directions be written in your own language at the pharmacy. If you speak a foreign language and your pharmacist does not, you may have to translate the directions into your written language for him so he can place the instruction on your bottle of pills. Nothing could be more frustrating than to have the medication you need on hand and not understand how to take it. Don't let them use the word "hypertension" instead of "blood pressure" if you don't know what the word hypertension means. Blood pressure is a common term almost everyone understands.

I also want to know the drug's possible side effects before I agree to try it or buy it. Feel free to ask whether your doctor has some professional samples you may try before buying a really expensive new medicine.

It becomes infuriating to pay a hundred dollars for a small handful of pills only to learn later that your body cannot tolerate the side effects or they cause an allergic reaction.

REMEMBER: Some allergic reactions to medications and/or environmental factors are life threatening in the extreme. This reaction is called anaphylactic shock and you may die quickly if an antidote is not readily available.

If you know you are allergic to ANYTHING this life threatening, wear an alert bracelet at all times that tells medical personnel about it. Most medical facilities and personnel are now trained to look for these medical emergency messages on your wrists. Wearing one could save your life.

How does your doctor or nurse practitioner—a fairly new medical professional field—decide from among a handful of possible medications, just which one will work best for you to restore your body to health?

I also want to know what harm this medication can do to me and how this can be counteracted. Is it safe if I take it with other prescribed or over the counter (OTC) supplements and herbs that I am using? Be truthful with your health care provider about ALL prescription medicines and herbal supplements you may be taking.

Some prescription medications were formulated from the same plants the herbals were made from, so if you are combining some, you may be accidentally overdosing.

Give your health care provider a list of your current medications and supplements or better yet, take the bottles with you when you go for an office visit. Ask, "Why is this particular medicine you are prescribing for me better than the older tried and true models? Why should I pay $15 per pill when there is a ten-cent generic variety that has been on the market for scores of years? How is this one better?"

New medications are being formulated and marketed every day, and some are really both necessary and better for you, but some of the older versions are still very effective.

Several new drugs have been on the market for as little as two years, and in wide general use, when several in the user population began dying as a result of the medicine before it got recalled by the drug makers. Remember Vioxx and Bextra? There have been others but those two are the most recent recalls I can remember. If you have to pay the entire cost for these new medications without insurance reimbursement, this can be quite a drain on your budget so generic medications or older formulations for your problem may be all you can afford and you should advise your doctor of that fact.

Sometimes the doctor's nursing staff can help make those expensive medications available to you by contacting a drug company to get the drug at greatly reduced or no cost to you. Some states and now Medicare Part D have drug prescription plans that provide drugs at a discount. Do not be afraid to ask for assistance. Remember, it is better to have some type of older medication than not to have any at all. Be honest with your provider and ask questions.

Does your doctor accept new medication samples from drug company representatives and pass those free samples to his patients? This act should be outlawed. The drug representatives should not be allowed to enter doctor's office to leave samples. This only tempts the doctors and nurse practitioners to prescribe this new medicine which may or may not be any better than what you already are taking. In return for their prescribing them to their patients, the health care professionals may be compensated by the drug's makers.

Passing out free samples is good in one way and bad in another. For those who absolutely cannot afford to buy a prescription, freebies can be very useful. But freebies also offer a very high temptation to some nurses who may be low on cash, to give them to friends for some type of payment. Thankfully, this type of crime is very low.

Perhaps it would be more efficient to place these drug samples in the druggist's hands instead of the doctor's office staff. Druggists would be an independent qualifier of whether or not you needed the free meds. And I believe since they would be in every drug store, there would not be the incentive to snag you as their customer. You could be anyone's customer since they all would offer the same service without their having to fill out and maintain mounds of paperwork on you as the doctors are required to do. The pharmacist would, however, need a written prescription from your doctor before dispensing these free meds. But you could also look at freebie pills as the doctor's way of acquiring and keeping you as his patient.

If your doctor always prescribes the most expensive new drug on the market—unfortunately some do—and offers you free samples, you might ask if drug companies pay them for prescribing the drugs. Don't be shy, ask the hard questions.

Many drug company representatives have only a half dozen medical practices they call upon on a regular basis, but they have several thousand dollars worth of rewards for those offices which prescribe their pills.

Both you and I have seen sad-eyed senior citizens nearly crying on television ads about their expensive medications and how desperate they are to get help to pay for them. They never seem to feel the urge to doubt whether or not they really need them to begin with. These senior citizens in ads are **COMPENSATED** by the drug companies but they can really play on your emotions. The nation's drug companies are spending billions of advertising dollars to lure today's susceptible aging generation

into a doctor's office to be prescribed their new drugs.

The current health care biggie on television is for the sale of motorized scooters for the elderly. The gray beards sing their praises of these little git-mobiles in those ads. Medicare will buy one for you for better mobility if a doctor prescribes one. It might be better if Medicare would just pay the fees for these seniors to enter a water aerobics class to gain mobility in that manner. That way at least the mobility gained would be permanent.

Older seniors that I am more personally familiar with will also tell you sadly how sick they are. "It's my heart, I need a new one," they might tell you with a long face as they thump their hand on their chest and then whip out a massive list from their wallets of their medications the doctor had given to them.

They carry this list with them at all times and compare it to their friend's list which might contain an even longer list of medications. These lists are more entertaining than grandchildren's pictures for some of these folks. "I am really sick, I need all these pills just to get by," one sadly told me. I nearly cried listening to him.

Does anyone really need this many medications or are more and more of our senior citizens being over-medicated? Do the doctors remove some older medicines when they add new ones? Are they making it clear to their patients that the older medicines should be discontinued and make sure that order is understood? I sure hope so but I doubt it in some cases.

When a friend died at age 50 from complications of diabetes he was taking more than 27 pills and insulin shots every day. From the time he was diagnosed until he died about 12 years later, the doctor did not discontinue a single pill from his daily drug cocktail. He moved like a zombie. I have seen and known others just like him.

Another senior I know measures how sick she is by how much her medications cost her. The more they cost, the sicker she must be, she will tell you. She never thinks about whether or not they improve her quality of life, but how much she had to spend to buy her medicine. She is a sincerely dedicated hypochondriac and sees her doctor or visits the local emergency room at least two or three times every week for her imaginary illnesses. She is 83 years old and dances three nights every week. Does she need medication? I doubt it. She has twice told me her doctor had told her she had "ridiculitis" and had given her pills that cost $92 for a 5-day supply, yet to her she was sick with a very painful illness. Is this "mind over matter?" Perhaps but it was fed by her doctor.

If she has a perceived reaction to the medicine or she simply does not like it for one reason or another, she dumps her $100 pills down the toilet. What a waste.

Also, many drug company ads on television will use well-known aging movie stars that we seniors grew up loving, trusting and watching all our lives to promote their latest products. These actors who may have never actually used the drug themselves that they are touting are **COMPENSATED** for their endorsements by the drug companies to extol their value. This disclaimer may or may not show up in very small print at the bottom of the ads. Of course most of us believe every word they tell us. Surely someone we have "known" so long would not lie to us. Would they?

All such ads will tell you at their conclusion to "ask your doctor if this medication is right for you." So, we senior citizens march right into our doctor's face during the next visit and ask just that. Knowing that they also will be rewarded handsomely for prescribing this medicine, our doctors agree and whip out that little prescription pad and start scribbling. They have been devoted drug company slaves ever since they received a drug company sponsored scholarship to medical school.

I am sure that most medical practitioners will not tell you whether or not they are compensated for prescribing a particular drug, but ask anyway. Sometimes you can tell by their reactions to your question if you were right on the mark.

I hate to go to my doctor's waiting room and sit for anywhere from 10 minutes to an hour while I wait to see the doctor even though I had a set appointment time. Then, while impatiently waiting, I see a drug company representative waltz in, nod at the receptionist who buzzes the door open so the agent can walk right in.

That agent is taking up the time you are paying for. You obviously had an appointment for a certain time slot, the agent did not.

There has to be a better means and a better time for the drug agents to make contact with the doctors. Perhaps they could all get together and hold a drug fair three or four times a year so the agents could explain their new products and give out samples to the doctors at that time. Then on a regular basis, more free samples could be mailed to the doctor's office or alternately dropped off at drug stores for distribution to the ailing patients thereby eliminating one huge problem and annoyance.

Death-Defying Acts

About fifteen years ago I started having extreme pain in my lower back. Nothing I took relieved this crippling pain which became more agonizing with each new day.

My problem started in February of 1992 while I was on a trip to Spain to see our older son and his family. I noticed while I was sitting in that tiny little seat on the airplane that pain was becoming a real problem for me.

I spent about three weeks with my son and found out when my plane took off to bring me home that after two hours of sitting still that I had to stand up. The pain was so severe the stewardesses let me stand in the galley with my back pressed firmly against the bulkhead. I was nearly paralyzed with pain. It was so bad I even offered to bail out over Chicago and take a cab home.

Arriving home I immediately got an appointment with my doctor who recommended that I see an orthopedic surgeon. I did so and she ran X-rays, MRIs, CT scans and whatever else was needed to determine what my problem might be.

She found that my tailbone had all but fallen off and decided it was probably a genetic problem when she learned from me that my mother's had done the same thing. Every move I made, whether it was simply breathing, caused that loose tailbone, or more properly named coccyx—to rotate and cut through the muscles of my lower back.

Because I am heavy she recommended we wait until the fall months to do the surgery to cut down the risk of infection. I agreed, but by the middle of September that year I just could not stand the pain any longer so she scheduled the surgery to remove this bone in October.

The surgery went fine and I was released the next day after being given intravenous infusions of antibiotics and morphine for pain for 24 hours. I made it home, barely, before giving in to grief for the absence of this part of my anatomy. The pain was still excruciating; where was the morphine now?

The surgeon had found that I needed over a hundred stitches in my back muscles to repair the damage done by the rotating sharp-edged coccyx so the surgery was far more extensive than either she or I had expected.

Three months later I woke with a very painful backside with massive drainage which indicated to me there was an infection present.

I had served as a volunteer emergency medical technician on the local ambulance service for ten years. I was properly trained and registered by both the state and national medical licensing boards so I had a pretty good knowledge of anatomy and diseases due to this excellent training.

I called the doctor's office and explained my problem to the office personnel. She passed my comments to the doctor who called me to say, "There is no infection. It has been just over three months since I did the surgery so it is time the stitches were absorbed. You had so many stitches inside that your body could not absorb them all so it is expelling the remainder of them," she advised. "Keep tissues back there to absorb any moisture. You can expect this to happen again before you are truly well," she explained.

I tried to tell her there was more than "moisture" back there but she still refused to make an appointment for me to see her.

Time went on and it happened two or three more times. I dealt with it.

In July of 1993, my husband and I went on a fishing trip to Lake Michigan. The water was rough that day, but we decided to try to do a little fishing near the shore anyway. I had been feeling fine up until the water got rougher. Our boat went way down into a deep trough of water and hit bottom with a bang which sent me straight up in the air about a foot off the cooler I had been seated on.

When I was slammed back down on the cooler I felt something flash from my wounded backside. When my husband looked, there was blood up almost to my neckline in the back. The roughness of the water had ruptured the incision.

We immediately returned home and I called the surgeon's office and demanded that she examine me. The office assistant finally agreed and the next day I was permitted to enter the inner sanctum.

The doctor took one look and said, "Oh, my, we are going to have to go back in there and redo everything. You have had a fistula form back there."

I explained that I had been trying for several months to get back in to see her with no success. "I could not get past the dragon in your outer office," I told her. She was not in the least sympathetic.

To shorten this story I was readmitted to the same hospital where the original surgery had been performed for the removal of this new fistula and to tighten up the incision again. The next morning after this second surgery I woke to find I could no longer use my left leg. It was now swollen enormously, painful to the point of my considering suicide, and it would not obey my mind's commands. I could only drag it behind me. The right leg had to do everything.

I went back to the surgeon again, this time on crutches and she asked why I was using them.

"That is the only way I can get around," I explained. "Well, how long has it been this way," she asked.

I replied that it had started the day after the second surgery and I said I thought she had caught a nerve or something, because the pain was exquisite and escalating but she said that was impossible to happen.

"It is just that you have developed chronic arthritis. Go back to your regular doctor and see what he can advise," she said.

I immediately drove across town to see my primary care doctor. He sat me up on the examination table with my legs dangling down for several minutes and then measured the swelling in my legs. The left leg was an inch and a half larger than the right one.

"You have arthritis," he told me. "Go back to Doctor X; she is the best in town."

I still didn't believe they were correct because I had had no arthritis one day and the next day I was suddenly immobilized with it after undergoing this surgery. But it is very difficult to argue with two trained doctors when you are hurting so badly.

The surgeon took a big needle and stuck cortisone right into the left knee joint. This permitted me to drive home and I was pain-free for eight days. Then the pain was back with a vengeance. Two doctors whom I had trusted said I had arthritis and initiated treatment for it without running a single test other than to measure the swelling in the legs. I later learned there are specific things they can check and tests that can be made to determine if you have arthritis.

A rheumatologist I finally consulted privately said I didn't have arthritis at all. After an MRI of my legs he said I had torn the cartilage in my left knee trying to walk by dragging the leg because of the pain I had been experiencing. The right knee also showed extensive damage because it had been doing the work of both legs. He recommended knee replacement surgery which I declined.

Then three months after this second surgery I awoke one morning running a very high fever and with an enormous abscess in the left lower abdomen and groin area.

The surgeon who finally operated on it explained that it was about ten inches long, and went eight inches deep down into my body.

"I have never seen an infection or an abscess this large," he and several of the hospital's nursing staff told me. He asked me if I minded if on his daily rounds he brought interns to my room to view this ugly mess and to educate them on the problems of sepsis. I agreed, thinking maybe it would help others.

The first morning when I had noticed this abscess at home I told my husband, "I have a nine down here. I can lie on my seven but I can't lie on my eight," as I pointed to my right and left sides and groin area.

He didn't have the foggiest idea what I was trying to tell him but I thought I was being very clear about the whole thing. I was apparently incoherent from the beginning of this latest medical problem but neither my husband nor I recognized that fact.

I took an antibiotic I had left over from another infection and two ibuprofen tablets and went back to bed. I could neither eat, drink, or use the bathroom.

This went on for three days, every four hours around the clock I took more medication and went back to bed before my husband finally realized there was something grossly wrong with me. He took my temperature and found it was just over 104 degrees and decided I was going to the hospital or doctor immediately.

We called my primary care doctor, the same one who had measured my "arthritic leg," so I could be admitted to the hospital. I figured since I had been seeing him for the past twelve years or so that his office was the correct place to start in getting myself admitted to a hospital.

My husband and I knew there was something gravely wrong inside my body but we both made a gross error in calling my primary care doctor as we would learn. But at the same time, we were attempting to do the right thing for me.

We called his office prior to leaving home and learned he was not in his office that day. His nurse called him to ask if he could come in and see me and he agreed so we met him at the office. Upon arrival at his office he pulled on a long white doctor's coat that had been hanging there on a peg in the hallway and came into the exam room. I was lying there already stretched out and I watched him pull on this white coat.

I have no idea how many times the coat had been worn previously, but it could have been worn several times or weeks for that matter. Each time it was worn he could have picked up more germs from his other patients before I encountered him.

Taking one look at my problem he said baldly, "You are toxic and septic. You need immediate surgery or you are going to die."

I believed him. I knew I was gravely ill so I agreed to go to the local teaching hospital for surgery.

Then, contrary to all my expectations, this doctor—who was a hulking six and a half footer and perhaps 275+ pounds—pulled my left leg off the table and held it there with his big belly.

Without asking my permission or saying a word to me or providing for any type of life support or anesthesia for me he picked up a scalpel and slashed into this abscess. Once he had cut it open, he started squeezing against the abscess with all his strength.

It had been so sore I could not touch it and I had padded it against being touched even by my softest loosest clothing, now he was squeezing it tightly in his meaty hands.

At that point in his treatment I lost all reason and started screaming for help.

I was so weakened by the sepsis when it hit my brain that I could not fight him off even though I tried. I remember trying to push and hit him away from me, but I was too limp and weak by then to be effective.

I am convinced that I felt the sepsis hit my brain as soon as it hit my bloodstream that day. The doctor ordered his nurse to cover the wound he had made with an un-sterile exam gown since it was the largest blotter they had on hand and I was bleeding and draining profusely.

He then went out to the waiting room and asked my husband to help the nurse "package me" for transport to the hospital in our car. Although it was only a mile or so to the hospital, he said, "We cannot wait for the ambulance, she could die before it gets here."

This was not good news. My husband told me later there were two men seated in the waiting room with him and when I started screaming they literally ran from the office, probably never returning to see this doctor.

The doctor sat at his desk almost feverishly calling other doctors to take over my care. I finally was able to remind him of the name of the surgeon who had removed my gallbladder several years prior to this and whom I liked and trusted, so he called him. The surgeon agreed to take over my care. That was the last time I ever saw this primary care doctor or spoke to him.

Always, prior to this time, when I was hospitalized while I was his patient but had been referred to a surgeon, he called and came by my hospital room each day to check on me even though a surgeon was over my care. But after this major blunder; he never again made contact with me nor I with him.

I believe that he panicked when he saw such a huge abscess and realized what a mistake he had made in trying to operate on me in his office.

He was nearly having a heart attack as my husband wheeled me past him in a wheelchair to our car. The doctor had made a huge blunder with me by cutting that abscess open and I believe he realized it. I have heard that he has since died.

Later a cousin of mine who speaks really soft and slow would tell me, "Helen, you tell your husband that the next time you start talking of sevens, eights and nines, he should just remember these numbers, nine-one-one." (Good advice).

On that fateful day while I was being driven to the hospital by my husband, the doctor called the emergency room and told them I was being brought in and that I was in critical condition. He explained to them that this surgeon was taking over my care, but to admit me to the intensive care isolation ward in the meantime. They were waiting for me and immediately started working to stabilize me.

I was admitted to the hospital and for the next two weeks I lay there completely at their mercy. I was placed on an electric ice blanket in an attempt to lower my temperature which was more than 103 degrees by the time I had gotten admitted. On my front side was a hot pad to try to drain the abscess.

I was told by the nursing staff that when one has sepsis it normally causes an abscess on one of the body's vital internal organs such as the heart, liver or a lung so I was sent for whole body scans. But the only abscess I had was the one visible on my left side which was shown to involve my left ovary, bladder, left kidney and the lymph nodes to my left leg as well.

Over the next fourteen days I would have almost 200 bottles of intravenous antibiotics and other liquids pushed into my system, and my temperature would soar just over or occasionally just under the 105 degree mark. My brain was quickly being burned up.

I ended up with no short-term memory, was bedfast for many months and for several years I sometimes had to use a wheelchair as a result. I also had to undergo eight years of on-again, off-again physical therapy to obtain even a modicum of my former mobility. I constantly exercised my brain during this time working crossword puzzles, cryptograms and other mind games to counteract the damage done by the drugs and fever. My brain is now about 90% recovered but that is more than I ever expected to recover. My physical recovery is no more than about 60 percent.

While I was in the hospital, I was taken to the water treatment room twice daily where I was lowered into a long trough of tepid water by means of a hydraulic trapeze. Once I was sitting in this tepid water secured by that same trapeze the whirlpool was turned on and they scooped in a dozen or so big scoops of crushed ice. I was made to stay in the water until my fever and the water's motion melted the ice then I was removed, rebandaged and taken back to my room. But nothing they did could lower my temperature.

Finally after undergoing additional major surgery and the doctors telling my husband to call in my family if they wished to visit me one more time, I started getting better. Prayer had worked when nothing else had and I decided I would live so I started fighting harder for my life. All the time I lay there my husband was faithful about visiting every day even though it was freezing cold outside because of a deep snow on the ground and he had to drive an hour each way to get there. He bathed me and washed my long matted curly hair which was driving me to distraction.

He also mopped my floor, cleaned my bathroom, emptied my trash and used bleach on everything in sight.

It got to the point that when the nurses saw him coming down the hallway they started gathering up the cleaning supplies they knew he would ask for.

Spreading Germs

I learned while lying there helpless in that hospital bed that a hospital is both the absolute worst place and the best place to be for the very ill person.

It is the worst place if you are already sick because it is filled with the germs of previous patients whose presence can never truly be eradicated. You sometimes go home from the hospital with deadly or infectious germs (MRSAs) you have gathered while in there for another, perhaps minor problem.

It is the best place because you can get tests, scans and treatments there that you could never get at home or in a limited nursing facility.

I also learned how germs are spread in hospitals and trauma centers where body fluids are common. To this day it nearly makes me sick to my stomach to recall some of the things I saw nurses do who should have known better.

My first and second shift nurses were pretty nice overall. The head of nursing on the third shift was the original version of Nurse Crachett portrayed in the movie, "One Flew Over the Cuckoo's Nest" fame. It is nurses like her who permit and encourage the infestation and spread of germs in hospitals. This nurse always arrived in my room already gloved even though there was a box of clean gloves hanging in every room.

How many patients had she seen and touched while wearing that same pair of gloves? There is no way of knowing. She was protecting herself, but she was spreading germs from patient to patient.

When she bandaged my side she put the barest minimum of padding on it so for her entire eight hour shift I was always wet, stinky and uncomfortable. It was like she was trying to save on supplies or something.

She repeatedly told me how expensive these supplies were and she also knew I had no health insurance so maybe she was trying to limit the hospital's losses.

One night while she had been applying a new bandage on me I asked if she would bring me some fresh ice water before she went back to her desk. I was so thirsty from all the fever that I was nearly dying.

After she was finished with the bandaging she grabbed my pitcher in her gloved hands, and went to the ice machine in the hall, dipped in with that pitcher and brought it back to my bathroom where she put fresh water in it and placed it back on my bedside table.

Only afterwards did she remove her gloves (hot with germs and disease from her patients) and place them in my bathroom trashcan. ONLY AFTER she had been in the communal ice chest with gloves on that had treated and come into contact with bio- hazard bodies like mine did she do this. I swear this is true because I watched her.

Every one of the seven patients in my sector was expected to die according to one of my male duty nurses who accidentally told me this news.

The actions of that one third-shift nurse may be one reason for our possible demise I later thought. Another incident I remember with this same nurse was one night she had helped me to the bathroom. I could not take a single step alone without collapsing to the floor so someone always had to assist me.

Because of my allergic reaction to tape, it could not be used to hold the bandage in place. Instead, they used an elasticized fabric stocking up my body to hold the bandaging in place. While I was sitting there on the throne that night my bandage fell off onto the floor.

I buzzed the nurse and told her she would have to bring more bandages because this one had fallen onto the floor.

"Just pick it up and place it back on," she advised me over the intercom.

An aide heard us, came to the bathroom and helped me back to my bed and then re-bandaged my wound with clean sterile bandages.

It wasn't many nights after this that I rang for this nurse and told her I needed to use the bathroom for a bowel movement.

She kept saying, "I'll be there soon." I rang several more times and her answer was always the same, "I'll be there soon," but, sadly, her "soon" was not soon enough.

I finally had to buzz her back and tell her she was too late but could she please come and help me clean myself up again. Perhaps she was punishing me, or maybe to give her credit she just forgot me, but she never answered that buzzer.

I would not see her for the rest of that night and I went back to sleep on dirty sheets and wearing a soiled gown.

The next morning when the day shift nurses came on duty I was still lying in my own—by then dried—defecated mess. They were horrified and asked how long I had been lying in that mess. I could only answer truthfully, "since about 3 a.m."

You must understand that I was totally helpless during this entire two-three weeks. I hated having to be dependent upon someone else to take care of my most basic bodily functions, and although it was embarrassing, I had no choice. There are many patients like myself in our hospitals today.

The following is another example of how germs are spread. On a day shift the first week I was there the nurses gave me a bath and placed me in a chair while they remade my bed with fresh linens.

While sitting there I leaned forward slightly to reach for my hairbrush and when I did that a huge abscess ruptured and I started bleeding profusely. I stood up on the sheets that had been removed from my bed and thrown to the floor at my feet.

The upholstered chair was quickly soaked with this rotten discharge by the time I could stand up. Close to a pint of dead liquefied body fluid flowed from my body and onto this fabric upholstered chair and then down onto the dirty sheets.

One of the nurses who had been making my bed ran into the bathroom and vomited when she smelled the stuff. The other ran from the room and got a bottle of squirt disinfectant for necrotic (dead tissue) odors.

Shaking badly by then, I apologized for the stink but they understood and explained that this is what happens when the body starts to decay and they took care of the mess.

But instead of removing the chair for a thorough cleaning, they merely used the already damaged bloody sheets and wiped the stuff off the chair as best they could; the remainder stayed on it and dried—perhaps becoming transparent—but still there nevertheless. **From that time on, when anyone visited me, I had them go into the hallway to the linen trolly and bring back a clean sheet to place over that chair before they sat down.**

The hospital I was in when all this happened to me always sends me a questionnaire after I have been discharged and at home for awhile to get my reactions to the quality of my care.

I replied with my complaints about the one night nurse and they advised me that she had already been discharged. It seems my first shift nurses believed what I had told them about her and had taken my complaints to management when she had neglected to clean up my night mess. Management had already acted by firing her. It would be interesting to know where she is working now.

Perhaps if you are hospitalized and you have a tall, thin nurse who, when she leans over your bed looks like a vulture, you know where she might be working now.

She is the only person I ever knew who could wear a turtleneck sweater with the entire neck part turned straight up and still have neck left over before her chin started. She wore a turtleneck sweater every night under her uniform top.

I was but one of that hospital's thousands of patients that year. How pervasive was this lack of cleanliness? Is this typical of the industry? I do not know, but I read admonitions in the newspapers and magazines every day about this very same thing and about hospital borne super germs. It is really scary but totally believable from my personal experiences.

Another hospital I have been taken to several times in the last five years due to injuries from falls I have had became another big problem for me. It missed several times in finding out what had brought me to their facility.

This hospital was closer than the one I have described above but it missed a simple broken leg; it missed finding a huge blood clot in my left groin area that almost killed me. I was in this particular hospital because I thought I had pneumonia and bronchitis. They found that ailment easily but missed why I was holding my left groin area tightly and screaming in pain.

The antibiotics cleared up my lung problem but my groin area was not even looked at. I left that hospital still holding my left hand in the painful area and screaming in pain to go home.

Two days later my personal doctor sent me to a rural hospital in his town. Within less than 5 minutes in the MRI machine, my problem was found. I had this huge blood clot and they immediately airlifted me to a city hospital for immediate surgery to remove it. Three days after that I awoke to no pain and learned I was in the critical ward. I had been in a coma for 3 days and knew nothing of what had occurred.

Not long after returning home from this incident I fell while I was outside in my lawn, onto frozen ground under a layer of melted snow and ice. I was taken by ambulance back to this hospital that missed the blood clot for X-rays. They found no breaks anywhere on my body, decided to wrap my ankle in two turns of an elastic bandage and sent me home, crying with pain.

When a couple days passed and the pain was still almost unbearable, my doctor sent me back to the other local hospital to be X-rayed again. I had broken not only my right leg, but two toes, another foot bone, my right thumb and my right shoulder which needed corrective surgery and involved me being in a padded sling for 13 weeks. The CEO of that first hospital was not interested in hearing my complaints. My husband had been on our way to celebrating the removal of my left leg cast and boot one day earlier by going out to supper. The two of us spent hours in a hospital that didn't seem to care they missed diagnosing my six bone breaks in one fall.

Once I had been diagnosed with Type II diabetes, I was advised by my doctor to see my eye specialist for a checkup. I was examined by the doctor, picked up the prescription and took it to Wal-Mart Vision Center to have it filled. A few days later I came down with the worst case of pink eye my doctor had ever seen. It took approximately three weeks and several different types of medicated eye drops before we saw any improvement.

He would tell me the following year that, "I wish I had taken a picture of your eyes. A friend told me I looked like a "she devil" my eyes were so brightly and totally red. They were a good textbook example of pink eye. You had it worse than anyone I have ever seen."

But since I was still almost non-mobile from my other hospital experiences, I was only in his office and Wal-Mart. I contacted Wal-Mart about having their greeters wash down the cart handles with a disinfectant prior to pushing them out to the public thinking that I had contracted my infection from those cart handles which are covered with all manner of germs.

But the mystery was solved the following year inside my trusted eye doctor's office when he told me how bad mine had been and added, "We had more cases of pink eye last year than I could ever remember having."

I had entered his office for my annual exam and his assistant asked me to place a hand-held eye blackout device in front of first one eye then the other. She made some evaluation from this and wrote it on my chart and placed the device back inside a drawer. I believe I contracted pink eye from this simple device since Wal-Mart declaimed having any other pink eye patients. The assistant assured me when I asked how often the device was cleaned, that it was cleaned after every use, yet she had just placed it back into the drawer without cleaning it after I used it. This explained the mystery of the pink eye epidemic to me to my satisfaction.

Surgeon's Report

I was seeing the same surgeon again a few years after the above incident for a minor surgical matter and he remembered me and my sepsis problems very well.

Since none of the tests they ran on me while I was incapacitated that time showed which of the germs was causing my problems I inquired of him what he thought the germ could have been.

"Well, we cannot be positive, but I treated you as though you had e-coli," he informed me.

The test results were all negative, nothing from my body would culture, yet I had been lying there in that hospital bed near death from infection.

"Had you had other surgery or been hospitalized prior to becoming this sick," he asked me.

I replied that I had had back surgery only three months prior and he exclaimed, "That's it, I'll bet you picked up e-coli from your hospital room."

Had I been sleeping in the same bed used previously by an infected patient that had not been cleaned properly? It is possible. Or, the germs could have been on the hands or instruments used in my surgery. We will never know at this point. This surgeon said the reason nothing would culture was because I had taken the oral antibiotics at home prior to coming to the hospital.

"BUT, if you had not taken them, you would be dead. There is no doubt about that. But because you did take them you are alive, so we will never know exactly what you had."

I learned from him that the mortality rate for having sepsis is 75-80%. Both my parents' cause of death was listed as sepsis.

Mother died in another hospital after gallbladder surgery; Dad died in a nursing home with several bed sores on his body. I was luckier than they. I was younger and stronger but sepsis still nearly took me out of this world.

That infection is not to be trifled with. It is deadly and can quickly kill you.

Perhaps the male night nurses helped save my life or the young nurses' aide who rebandaged me when my bandage landed on the floor. I am seeing more and more male nurses when I am admitted to the hospital and I'm glad they are entering the health care arena. The ones I have encountered are excellent providers. It does not embarrass them to do the worst and nastiest chores even though it is embarrassing to the patient to have to ask one to do the nasty in cleaning their bodies after using the bathroom. I'm convinced these young men will make wonderful nurses. I have now encountered them in three or four of the hospitals I have been admitted to. They are terrific.

One of my doctors I have visited for years was hopeful that the first hospital I spoke about and others like it could find a spray antiseptic that could be opened in every room between patient admittances that would kill every germ in that room in less than five minutes. I'm hopeful also. He said to me, "Have you ever seen them wash the bed down while you were being dismissed? Yes. Did you see them wash the rails down? No. They change the sheets and remake the bed between patients, and empty the trash. It looks clean, but from my own experience and the experience of this one podiatrist I had visited for about 40 years, had not seen them clean and wash a bed down either. Two of my surgeons refused to admit their patients to the hospital in the nearby town where I was admitted for sepsis because of the bad outcome their own patients received.

There has now been a brand-new hospital built completely across town and the one I was in with sepsis and other problems earlier in life has been town down to the bare earth and all the surrounding buildings affiliated with that hospital have met a like fate and are gone. The only thing left on that lot is the parking garage and the entire acreage, including the parking garage, is now surrounded by an eight-foot-tall heavy chain link fence.

There is a picture elsewhere in this book of the two hospital locations. The new one that was opened about a year ago looks like something from Star Wars it is so modern and huge. I just hope it stays cleaner than the old one did.

As a result of my writing the first issue of this book, I sent the book to several hospitals where I knew a few of the people. The small rural farm town hospital did more than the big city hospitals have done to clean up the place. I'm glad the little I have learned might help others in my shoes later down the road.

I have watched toddlers trying to get up into the waiting room chairs in hospitals, with their little faces right down on the edge of the dirty, probably germ-infested, cloth covered chairs while their mother held her phone in front of her and ignored the young ones. I advocate that all these close covered chairs be recovered with a non-permeable material that can be wiped down several times each day with a cloth dipped in cleanser that will protect the little ones. The farm hospital I cite above has now completed a large portion of this chore. How nice to think what I say is being listened to.

Also, the doctor who told me said this was a very important book that should be required reading of every health care professional.

I spend hours and hours at this computer writing each and every day. My work can be found on Amazon and ordered for a nominal fee. I am proud that my words might make a difference to the health care industry if enough people read it.

New Doctor Search

I was so scared of doctors by the last time I talked with this surgeon that I had not seen a regular doctor for about five years. He said with my history I must have a primary care physician and he gave me a list to choose from. He appreciated my trust in him, but said he could not be a primary care giver, he was a surgeon.

I looked them over, got his recommendations, and settled on a doctor in my home county. It was a woman doctor and I came to care for her very much. We had instant rapport and I initially felt she was competent.

But because I broke out with the hives really badly one time after she had prescribed some medicine for me I began to look askance at her too.

I had consulted with her for a problem I had, I can't recall what it actually was now, and she had prescribed a drug whose base ingredient is sulfa, an ingredient I have been allergic to all my life and she knew it.

My allergy alert labels were printed in red and stuck on the front of my folder.

The day I broke out with hives I called the mail order druggist we used and asked what the problem might be. He said, "You know, we have your allergy notices on file here. I saw that your doctor had prescribed this particular drug and that you were allergic to its main ingredient, so I called her.

She told me, "Give it to her anyway," he claimed as he apologized.

Another time I noticed I was having kidney problems. I had been told by the trusted surgeon to watch for any problems that might crop up as a result of my having had sepsis which sometimes damages one or more of the internal organs. And boy, have those organs been damaged!! It has been 30 years since I had sepsis and the final outcome is still not known. I survived the abscess the doctors told me was normal for this disease, but there no accounting for the damage it does to the internal organs, and the damage is vast. You never seem to outgrow that damage. It keeps coming back to haunt you even after 30 years.

In my case, it was the kidneys. In this instance, for unknown reasons, I started swelling and I could not urinate. No matter how much liquid I drank, I never felt the urge to use the bathroom.

This condition started on a Friday afternoon and by Monday morning I was desperate for relief but my doctor could not work me in until the next day her staff told me.

By the next day I was in the middle of congestive heart failure and my blood oxygen level was 79% which is a critical condition level I would learn later from reading a story in Reader's Digest. She gave me a shot in the hip to make me urinate and sent me home after telling me, "Now, you are a smart enough woman to know that if you don't get better or if you get worse, go on to the emergency room and tell them I said to admit you."

She was preparing to leave the next day for a medical conference, she said, and she would not be back in her office until the following Monday.

My doctor did not ask me to call someone to drive me home or order an ambulance to take me to the hospital that day. I was allowed to drive myself home with a critical lack of oxygen in my bloodstream. I could have fallen asleep driving, had a wreck and killed myself or someone because of this.

I am lucky I made it home safely without falling asleep at the wheel as I had done a few days earlier when I realized I was in trouble and needed medical attention.

Two days after my Tuesday appointment my husband came into the house and found me asleep and unresponsive in my chair. After much shaking and yelling, he finally roused me enough that I was able to walk to our car. That is the last thing I remember for three full days.

He drove me to the emergency room of this same hospital mentioned above where a catheter and a ventilator were inserted since my blood oxygen level was by then 57%, which was near fatal. I woke three days later to see a doctor (at least I assumed he was a doctor) leaning against the wall in the corner of my room reading my chart.

I had been on the phone when he arrived telling someone I was probably going to be discharged that day.

When he (I would later learn he was my assigned cardiologist) heard me say this he advised me, "Lady, we don't know yet if you are going to live or die. You are not going home today."

I asked him, "Do you mean I am really sick?" He assured me I was.

The funny thing was I didn't feel bad at all. I was kind of lethargic but I felt no pain. It was hard to think they had listed me in critical condition in their ICU once again. The ventilator had been stuck down my throat and every four seconds it would inflate my lungs so I could breathe for me.

I still believe if my primary care physician had admitted me to the hospital the day I went to see her then a lot of my problems during this episode could have been avoided. But she was in a hurry, planning to leave for the remainder of the week to attend a medical seminar, and I didn't have enough sense with my low oxygen level to push the right buttons and see that I got good medical care. My husband was busy with his business and did not realize my danger either.

But our young neighbor girl was an office assistant at my doctor's office and she recognized my danger. She kept telling my husband to take me to the hospital until finally he was convinced. But neither he nor I had any idea just how sick I really was.

Now, if I appear to be very sick, my husband goes to the doctor with me and I go with him. He, too, has learned to ask questions and demand quality care. We now support each other during office visits. (My husband has since passed away.)

Without having him as my medical advocate while I was in the hospital thirteen years ago, seeing that my body, bed, room and bathroom were clean and disinfected, I might not be alive today.

Since I started writing this book my husband had to have knee replacement surgery on his right knee.

We had been going to an arthritis specialist for almost two years with no good results to show for our efforts.

To begin with, this specialist would only recommend two places where he would recommend the surgery be done. Both were one to two hours away from our home and we both knew that was too far for me to have to drive to see him so began looking for another location to have his surgery done.

We immediately ruled out the hospital I had preferred to frequent due to its infection rate which continues out of control. We then looked at a hospital about 20 miles away but when we tried numerous times to call a specialist in that city we got one of those round-robin phones that never lets you talk to a human, so we ruled that one out. If the doctor was so busy even his nurses could not answer his phone we believed we would not like him anyway. Besides that, the hospital he practiced in was not very popular with us from being EMTs.

Looking further and after having asked several friends where they would recommend he be admitted we were referred to a really small community hospital, still only about 25 miles from home. We met with a new primary care doctor we now have who is attached to this hospital and he referred us in turn to an orthopedic surgeon in the same building.

We met with him, liked his manner, and questioned him about the rather small hospital where he practiced. He assured us it was a really nice hospital overall. Once my husband's surgery was behind us we could only agree with this surgeon's assessment.

My husband was given some medications to take to prepare for the surgery and he was taken off others for the same reason. About a week prior to his admission the hospital called and pre-admitted him over the telephone. They made arrangements for for my husband and me to meet with a group of people at the hospital the following week that would be responsible for his care.

I had never had this experience before, but it was wonderful and gave us a much better feel for this little hospital in a rural farm town.

At the meeting the next week we met with a patient advisor who went over every facet of his surgery with us. She performed an EKG, took his vitals twice, sent him to the laboratory for his pre-op blood work and gave him a device that was supposed to help his breathing during and after surgery.

In addition to all this she called in the anestheologist so the type of anesthesia could be determined beforehand. We also met with a physical therapist for 30 minutes and an occupational therapist for another 30 minutes. Wow, were we impressed? I should say we were. I was notified by telephone three times during and after his surgery and prior to their returning him to his room that everything was going as scheduled.

His surgery went off without a single hitch and within three weeks he was driving again. At the end of six weeks he was able to walk three miles in the wooded terrain to hunt for mushrooms. There was not a single incidence of infection or problems encountered during this whole time. In six months, the surgery was only a memory.

I tell you all this to illustrate what a little more care of the patient means to the hospital's users. Yet this same hospital is by far the smallest one we investigated. Why would his arthritis specialist not recommend a place that has this kind of record? All such centers could take lessons from these health care providers.

Other Advice

If you are fortunate enough to enjoy good health, take care of it. If not, there are some other precautions you should take.

Before you think you need a medical advocate (some refer to them as proxy's), make sure that you have appointed one in writing. I trusted my spouse to be mine. Perhaps you do also.

If you have no family members to rely on, then consider asking a good friend you would trust with your very life—because that is what you will be doing—to make good medical decisions for you if you are ever in the position I have been in twice during the past fifteen years. This person should be empowered to speak for you when you cannot speak for yourself.

This is not a duty to be granted or taken lightly. Chose someone you have absolute faith in and put your instructions to this person in writing, notarize it if necessary and keep it with you at all times and give your proxy a copy. You should give a copy to your primary care physician also so that he will know you have empowered this person to make your medical decisions and receive information on your progress if you become incapacitated. Take a copy with you to the hospital and put it on file there when you are admitted.

Without a medical advocate or proxy you are at the mercy of busy medical professionals who may pull your plug a little earlier than you would want it pulled.

Reiterating, I do not mean to imply that all medical professionals are uncaring people. Most of these people would give their very lives for their patients. For instance, my young neighbor who bugged my husband about how sick I was; she cared enough for me to make sure I got adequate attention. Or the people in the small rural hospital I described above.

One of the complaints I answered when queried by the hospital after my discharge was about their staff.

It has become popular with the medical professionals to have their office staff, from the registered nurses all the way down to the cleaning personnel, wear non-distinctive baggy, cutesy uniforms.

I have convinced myself that this became a common practice when the hospitals realized there was a shortage of nurses. If their patients could see all these uniformed people running around doing errands they would think the hospital was well staffed nurse-wise and be reassured.

I have learned this may not be the case at all. Half the staff you see bustling around hospital corridors could be custodial personnel or dish handlers for all a patient knows.

The once-proud registered nurses who in days of yore wore all white uniforms from head to toe, with a funny little white cap perched on her head, is now a thing of the past in a lot of health facilities. There might be only one RN on the floor of any hospital. There also may not be ANY RNs on the floor if the shortage is really as acute as some media stories report.

All those other busily scurrying bodies you see racing up and down the hall performing various errands in their cute little outfits could be cleaning personnel or kitchen helpers.

The RNs were once very proud to wear their distinctive white caps and uniforms. They worked hard and long and studied for years to earn that particular uniform. I think it is long past time to get back to a uniform in the hospitals that is distinctive for those with the most education and training.

The cleaning personnel or the lesser educated medical staff can wear the cutesy Pooh Bear costumes.

I would appreciate it very much though if the RN's wore their whites and the janitorial staff was designated by one standard color uniform such as blue or something, on an industry-wide basis, so I would know not to ask them about my medical condition. I also believe they are told to respond by saying, "I will tell your nurse what you need." They never admit to you that they are custodial or kitchen personnel.

So You Survived
and Made It Home

Once you leave the hospital you should ask for and pay to receive a copy of the charts that were maintained during your stay. These papers are in the hospital's archives and may be purchased for a fee. They are worth every penny you pay for them.

Some hospital patient charts are a complete work of fiction. I bought a copy of the charts from my 1992, 1993 and 2001 hospital stays. During my 1993 stay I lost 19 pounds which was good because I needed to lose weight, but it should also have indicated that I was not eating the food they placed in front of me three times each day. I sent that food back to the kitchen untouched primarily because it was poorly prepared and smelled like disinfectant.

Yet on my charts the nursing staff repeatedly wrote, "The patient was observed sitting up on the side of her bed enjoying her lunch, or dinner, etc."

I cannot remember for the life of me even being *able* to sit up alongside my bed without falling out of bed onto my head on the floor and I surely cannot remember eating their food. It was horrendous.

It was so bad that I got to the point of ordering chunks of cheese, fresh fruit, fruit juices, raw broccoli, boiled eggs, etc. that they could not destroy with their cooking methods and which did not have to be placed inside those insulated plastic dishes which reeked of dishwasher disinfectant.

Once I even accused them of bringing me a picture of a strip of bacon. You could pick it up, smell it, wave it around without breaking it, taste it, and still not know what it was you held in your hand. One breakfast I can recall I had ordered ham and scrambled eggs. When it arrived there was one piece of ham about the same size of a discarded fingernail snip in a couple of tablespoons of plastic eggs. I really think you could have bounced those fake eggs with your fork. Anyway, that entire meal was sent back to the kitchen.

And the little plastic insulated food containers and Styrofoam cups left a lot to be desired too. The plastic containers had been processed in the dishwashing detergents and sanitized so often they had absorbed that awful smell, ruining the flavor of any food served in them and the Styrofoam cups often collapsed, spilling liquids all over me since I was too weak to hold them securely.

If I ever am admitted into another hospital I fully intend to take my own small coffeemaker and glass mug with me.

Likewise the information gleaned from my body liquids they were supposed to monitor each time it left my body was mostly fabricated.

My night nurse would come in each morning and say something bright like, "How many CC's of urine did you do last night?"

I would reply that if she had checked it, wrote down the CC's of urine, and then emptied the overflowing pot each time I buzzed her as she was supposed to do, she would know the answer to her question. I was so sick I didn't even know what a CC was most of the time.

Yet she would write on my chart on the wall which became part of my permanent record, which I later purchased, that I had passed maybe 850 CC's of urine during the night.

As I said, some parts of those charts are pure fabrications and contain not a single grain of truth. Order a copy of your own charts and see just what I mean.

You must petition your health care personnel to write correct information about you on your charts.

If you tell your providers you are allergic to something, make sure they adhere to the written notices.

Never knowingly swallow a medication you know you are allergic to even though a nurse may say something like "Take this one pill and then we will call the doctor," as one once told me to do.

Tell her to call the doctor first because you are not going to swallow that pill. Your life may depend on this one little act of defiance.

One of my allergy notices most often violated includes the fact I am allergic to many of the tapes which are used by medical personnel. Even the lowly band-aids cause problems for me, yet every time blood is drawn from my arm, they immediately paste on a band-aid.

If I am wearing long sleeves and forget the band-aid is there for two or three hours, an infection sets in that takes months to heal. I don't think they will ever learn. I have gotten to the point where I won't let them apply one without reminding them of the allergy. If they still feel compelled to put one on me, I simply immediately remove it.

In conclusion, I just want to say be careful who you entrust your life to. Most health care professionals are just that, professional, but those few who are not can kill you.

What Should We Do Differently?

For starters we need better germ control in all areas of our medical care especially inside hospitals and our doctor's offices. Have you ever noticed that in all hospital rooms there is a fabric curtain on an overhead rail that can be pulled on and passed around a patient's bed to give the patient a little privacy?

That fabric is constantly being brushed up against by the nurses and doctors who have been brushing up against each of their patient's beds and bodies. This is one way that germs are passed.

The staff passes these germs which have collected on their clothing onto these curtains and the patients, in turn, then brush against the curtains, contaminating their bare butts each time this happens. And don't we all know and love how hospital gowns are designed?

In my own mind I have designed a pair of shorts that are opened and the patient placed on that open pair of shorts. The legs are then snapped closed around each leg with a hole in the groin for tubing to be placed in the bladder. The adjustable waist strap could be closed to fit. That would obliterate the need for an open backed gown that is 14 sizes too large for anyone to wear and cover our bare butts as we walk down the hallways.

Those fabric curtains need to be discarded in lieu of disposable paper ones which should be *replaced* between each patient admittance. That would eliminate one major source of constant contamination.

Disposable gloves in many size boxes are placed in every room. Use them!!! Do not go room to room with the same pair of gloves on the hands of our nurses. Use them properly, changing and disposing of used gloves before leaving the room or entering another room.

The entire room needs to be scrubbed and disinfected thoroughly between patients. I don't mean just run a damp mop over the floors and remake the bed with fresh linens. The walls, floors, bathrooms and beds should be scrubbed down with disinfectant. I have watched several times as the aides remade a fresh bed before I was even out of the room. I do not recall ever seeing them washing that bed itself or even the rails with disinfectant before replacing the linens or their cleaning the bathroom.

All fabric-upholstered furniture should be discarded from patient rooms because this furniture is full of germs. Sick people have sat on them as I did with that horrible discharge which was merely wiped down with a dirty sheet from my dirty bed!!

Not only that, but upholstered chairs in all waiting rooms are contaminated by fluid which leaks from people's bodies, especially sick ones. Many people are incontinent and this discharge is absorbed for those same chairs. All should be washable.

The visitor's chairs should be made of a material that will not absorb moisture and can be easily washed down with disinfectant. Then clean washable or paper slipcovers should be placed on the chairs between patient admittances and after such accidents as I had. This one act alone will protect both the patient while sitting in that chair and her visitors.

My podiatrist suggested to me there should be a germ killing aerosol can disinfectant developed that, once it is set off inside an empty patient room, could kill every germ on contact within five minutes of its use. He agrees with me about the germ-filled condition of the hospital where I was a patient.

When hospital rooms are being designed they should be engineered so the patient's naked behind is toward a solid wall, not toward the hallway as seems to be the norm in every room I have ever been in. This should be an easy fix in any new construction or major remodeling design.

No hospital should have its own cafeteria. Period.

The people in charge of the cafeterias have no idea what real food consists of nor do they know how to prepare it. If they must have a food service area, then let it be a dish-washing room and tray loading area only.

The food they serve their patients almost defies the definition of food. Sick folks need comfort food. Hospital personnel are not going to change the way we eat while having us as paying guests for only a few days, so why not give us something that makes us feel good when they prepare to feed us? Makes sense to me.

Food is such an important and very necessary fact of life and it is especially so for one recovering one's health.

All hospitals should build an auxiliary free-standing building to house a privately operated catering service. The license to cater the hospital's foods could be awarded to the best and most qualified bidder and their abilities should be re-evaluated prior to awarding any contract renewals.

The caterer should be allowed to serve food to hospital visitors, doctors and other workers to supplement their contracted earnings.

No insulated plastic containers should be used in food service. Only glass or ceramic dishes with one-time use plastic covers when needed should be used. And since we are usually there only a few days, perhaps I would allow pre-packaged plastic eating utensils, but stainless steel would be preferable.

The insulated plastic dishes taste exactly like the dishwasher detergents so should never be used.

The cold foods must be served cold and the hot foods should be served hot, even if this means having a microwave oven on every food cart to perform this magic.

If serving macaroni and cheese, it should be home-made using elbow macaroni and real cheese and not be made from a boxed national brand mac and cheese for example. The same goes for boxed mashed potato mixes. Give us the real thing or forget it.

Vegetables should not be cooked until they are an unrecognizable piece of mush on the plate. Instead, they should retain some crispness and look at least somewhat like their original state when served to the patients.

Serving stinky fish dishes in hospitals should be outlawed.

Fake eggs and white bread should be removed from all hospital food servings. It is so easy to make your own fake eggs using one whole egg and two egg whites, why use rubber eggs? Why not serve whole grain bread? Serving anything to a diabetic made from processed white flour is like giving them an overdose of medicine. It is bad for everyone.

Nurses who do not chart their patients or record fluid input/output correctly should be re-trained and if they still falsify the charts, they should be released from service.

These ideas might not be earth shattering to some, but implementing them would go a long way toward making our hospital admittances and patient recoveries more easily accomplished.

The medical associations are going to have to start monitoring the actions of all their members, especially the older ones, or those for whom they have received numerous complaints. Many of the older professionals fall victim to the same mental deficiencies we outsiders do. When it is determined their usefulness is nearing an end, they should be quietly and lovingly retired from service. This is an absolute must.

Protection of the patient has to come before any other consideration.

Implementing better cleanliness standards should go even further in preventing the growth and spread of hospital super germs. This is a must.

Protection of the patient has to come before any other consideration.

We are warned every day about these super germs which are becoming resistant to all known antibiotics. We need to be very careful.

A yearly report card of every health care facility in each state is a must. The report card I just read in newspaper stories about Indiana's hospitals listed about three dozen incidents where the patient was damaged by a doctor. Included were incidents—or errors as they were prone to call them—of removing the wrong limb, leaving instruments inside a patient and operating on the wrong organs as part of the report. This report does not include the number of patients who left the hospital and developed an abscess from a hospital-acquired germ. Those too should be made a part of every health care center's report card and it must be made available to the public.

Keep track of and report any excesses you become acquainted with to your own local health department and the state department of health. We can win this war.

Here's to your good health

Never Smoke Again

Going Cold Turkey:
How to Quit Smoking Forever

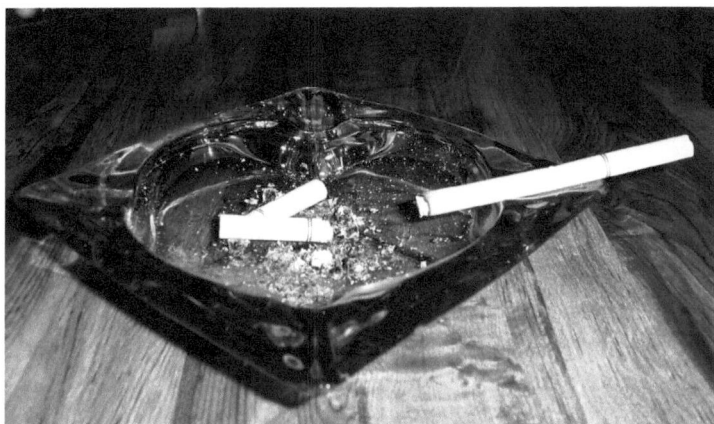

Let's Talk

I am going to teach you how to stop smoking and you will **never smoke again**. If you are a working stiff, then you need to schedule a week's vacation to begin this program; two weeks off would be better. But before I can do that I will try to help you determine why you use tobacco in the first place.

Do you smoke cigarettes because you like and want to? Or, does everyone you know smoke so you light one up also just to be sociable? Have you tried many times to quit and failed? Has your doctor prescribed medication, patches or gum to help you kick the habit? Are those aids stashed away in a dresser drawer somewhere, never used? Are you afraid you will gain weight if you stop smoking?

Once a friend of mine had proof read this manuscript she shared with me the fact that she was able to stop smoking on the advice of an old-timer who had told her she could do it if she followed the Zodiac signs. This is a successful way to stop also if you can figure out how to determine when the "signs" are in the knees. Careful reading of a current Old Farmer's Almanac will give you this information, but for some, the almanac is complicated reading. If it is for you, just ask any old timer in your neighborhood to advise you when the signs are in the knees. By the time the signs go out the feet, your nicotine craving will be gone.

Have you tried hypnotism or acupuncture only to walk out the door after a session to find yourself lighting up as you walked away from the building? I did that. Have you ever wondered what you would do with your hands when you are idle if you are not holding a cigarette between two fingers? Are you **READY** to quit?

Have you priced the cost of just ONE pack of cigarettes in recent years? What was about $2 a pack is now $10 a pack. How can you afford to pay this price just to damage yourself?

If you answered yes to any of my questions I will help you to **never smoke again.** Notice that I do not say I will help you to **TRY** to never smoke again. You will **never smoke again**, not just try to quit.

Do you like the way your clothes, cars and home **stink** because you are a smoker? Or, are you completely unaware how awful cigarette smoke smells to someone who actually can smell? I was at one time.

It does not matter how much fabric softener you use in your laundry to make your clothes smell fresher, or how much air freshener you spray in your home and cars. **They will stink** once they are exposed to your cigarette smoke!! You cannot hide the fact you are addicted to nicotine. It follows you around like a dark dust cloud, kind of like Pig Pen in the Charley Brown cartoons.

Do you realize that a non-smoker can smell your awful stink when they first get out of their car at your home? The stink is in the very air outside your home as well as inside. I promise I am telling you the truth.

Most people think, wrongly, that they cannot give up cigarettes. They have tried and tried to kick the nicotine habit but failed several times. I will admit it is a hard habit to kick. I will be the first one to say you are right on that score, **UP TO A POINT.** But I am here to also tell you it is **NOT AS DIFFICULT** as you might think **nor** is it **IMPOSSIBLE** for you to stop smoking for good.

Have you found yourself, more and more often in recent years, finding it difficult to maintain friendships or visit relatives or a favorite club or restaurant because they have all become smoke-free and you are still puffing away?

Are you one of those people who, in the cold months (and we have lots of those kinds of months in our Mid-West climate) huddle outside a door in the open-air, puffing away on a cigarette, no matter that it is coming a blizzard or pouring the rain outside. You huddle together like a football team before a scrimmage, perhaps barred and banned by city ordinances from smoking inside where it is warm.

So more and more often you sit alone at home where no one will be on your case about smoking, thinking you are happy, but you are really just depressed.

Some cities and towns have even banned throwing a lighted cigarette from your car's window because even though the ground is wet, it could torch and burn a walker!! You can be given a ticket in these areas.

Picture this: you are out of cigarettes, you cannot find even a long stub to re-light, and it is in the middle of a cold snowy night and the roads are slick and icy.

Have you found yourself bundling yourself and your kids into winter clothing, strapping the kids into their car seats where they will be safe, getting in the vehicle behind the steering wheel and setting out for an all-night convenience store to buy a pack of smokes?

You light up your first smoke as you leave the door of the convenience store and crawl into your still warm car.

You tapped that package against your opposite thumb pad several times, flipped your lighter and began puffing away on that beautiful cigarette. You crawled back inside your vehicle, blowing smoke all the while and your kids in the back seat begin coughing and you told yourself, deliberately wrongly, that they are coming down with a cold. **You know better than this!!**

In reality, they are not safe in their seats at all. They are held captive there by you so you can have that big satisfying puff, disregarding completely the fact that you are endangering their lives even more with your second-hand smoke. If this is you my friend, then you are truly addicted to that devil, nicotine.

What I Learned

I have found that most people need an excuse to smoke.

They say things like, "smoking calms me down, helps me to relax and keeps my weight under control. Smoking gives me something to do with my hands. I just like the taste of tobacco and I'll smoke as long as I want to and can afford them. People cannot tell me what to do or how to spend my money. If they pass a law banning cigarettes, I will find them somehow even if I have to grow my own tobacco."

I have heard people say all the above when supporting their addiction. I spoke a few of those excuses myself in my smoking days.

I'll tell you what I found out. I smoked because I thought no one cared about me. When I found out a lot of people loved and cared about me, I quit smoking **and never took another single puff**.

I didn't want to hurt the people I loved and who loved me.

You have to learn why you smoke.

Here's My Story

I awoke in a hospital's intensive care room one day, three days later than I remembered it being. Oxygen was streaming into my lungs from a machine beside my bed. A second machine was breathing for me every four seconds. I did not remember a thing that happened in the last three days. I had been comatose 3 days.

I was brought to the hospital's emergency room when my blood oxygen level was just 57%. I survived. The doctors could not believe it. It was almost unheard of for someone to survive with an oxygen level this low and not die or end up with brain damage. I was lucky and I know it.

The two cigarettes I smoked I had **lit at the same time** just before I left in the car for the hospital, and **which I don't even remember lighting,** were the last ones I have ever even touched. I **never smoked again** because when I woke up I was told by my loved ones how much I would be missed if I died. I never had a craving for a cigarette again. For me it was that simple.

For years I had been depressed without knowing that I was just because no one bothered to tell me they loved me. They would do nice things for me, but few ever said those three little, very important magic words to me. Finally someone told me they loved me and that was all I needed to hear. It turned my life around. Maybe you need to hear those words also. If you do, I'll say them now, **"I LOVE YOU."**

It took me 42 years of puffing on a pack and a half of cigarettes every day before I discovered that truth about myself. That is **613,200 cigarettes** that I smoked before I wised up. And that is a lot of cigarettes by anyone's standards. Measuring a cigarette at 4 inches long, that would mean I smoked the equivalent of a **38 mile long** cigarette!!!! Holy cow!!!

I **had** a very good friend, now deceased, who claimed he smoked five packs per day. I don't doubt that he did. And notice that I spoke in the **past** tense. He died of smoking related diseases when he was only 50 years old. His widow later died young also.

But multiply that number out. If he smoked the same number of years I did, and I'm sure he did, the count of his cigarettes was **1,530,000** cigarettes he smoked, the equivalent of a **72 ½ mile long** cigarette. **No wonder he is dead.**

You would think that by smoking that many cigarettes and dying at age 50, his wife would have been convinced to stop smoking, but she is still lighting up. I have another friend who has chronic obstructive pulmonary disease (COPD) who still smokes. Another loved one has asthma really badly, and she still smokes.

Why Should I Never Smoke Again?

Because if you do not stop smoking and **never smoke again** your chances of contracting lung cancer are astronomical. And yes, some non-smokers do get lung cancer. That excuse is no longer acceptable. But **most lung cancer patients have been smokers at some time in their life.**

Sadly some are so addicted to nicotine they even continue to smoke as they seek treatment for their terminal cancer.

Lung cancer is a very debilitating wasteful disease and it is painful, sometimes to the point of no relief. You generally have one or more surgeries to remove the tumors. Surgery is then followed by weeks or months of energy-draining sessions of chemotherapy and/or radiation treatments. If not detected very, very early (which is rare that it is discovered in this stage) your chances of survival are slim to none.

Your loved ones can only wait and watch you die by inches.

Often, the only answer is to die and so you do.

Your children are left without a parent, your spouse is now alone to carry on and try his or her best to keep the family together. Can you imagine how frustrated and just plain mad your surviving spouse would be if they had always been a non-smoker themselves? No matter how much you loved your mate, it was not enough, they loved the taste of tobacco more than they did you and now you are left to carry on alone.

Even worse would be if the one who died was the non-smoker and contracted lung cancer from your second-hand smoke. Would that convince you to quit smoking? Or if you kill your child with your second hand-smoke, would that convince you? You love your children and protect them by strapping them in a car seat when you drive and in many other ways, but all the while you are smoking around them in a confined space and they are breathing your second-hand smoke.

But lung cancer is the most easily preventable kind of cancer you can get. If you are not a smoker, please, don't start smoking. If you are a smoker you should quit and **never smoke again**. It is far easier to quit than you ever imagined it to be.

I believe our school systems are doing a good job teaching our children not to take up the smoking habit. I know my two sons learned the lesson well and pleaded with me for years to stop smoking. Why is it so hard for us, as adults, to learn the same lesson our children are taught in early elementary school?

That old demon nicotine can get hold of you and hang on tight. It is up to you to break the shackles and free your body from its ravages.

Smoking and inhaling tars and nicotine can make your body look 10 to 15 years older than your true age. It ages you much the same way drinking excessive amounts of alcohol does.

Your skin will have a sallow look, your face will be lined and wrinkled, and your fingers most likely will have the yellow stain of nicotine on them. It can decrease your libido. It can also affect your night vision when driving. Did you know that? It also causes a multitude of health problems other than cancer.

There is not one single health benefit to be gained by lighting up a cigarette.

So stop uttering excuses and just stop smoking. Lay that pack down and walk away. **Never touch them again.** It is not easy, but it is doable.

How Do I Never Smoke Again?

You have tried nicotine gum, pills, patches, willpower, hypnotism, threats. There are some people on which these aids work, but they did not work for me. Nothing has ever worked before but it will work now. You just need to be motivated to stop.

You will **never smoke again** if you follow what I have learned about successfully quitting smoking.

The night before you are going to quit smoking you should gather all your smoking paraphernalia together and dispose of it. Take all the cigarettes you have on hand and put them in the garbage. Then rid your home of that garbage so you cannot sift through it the next day looking for those cigarettes or long butts.

You empty, wash or dispose of all ashtrays. You empty and wash all your trash cans. You put the lighters or matches in proper containers and then you dispose of all these items permanently.

You will never need these items again, I promise you.

Go to bed and get a good night's sleep because tomorrow you are going to appreciate feeling rested.

Then What?

When you rise the next morning go into your bathroom and look in your mirror. What you see is the **old you**. When you quit smoking, you **will never see** that reflection again.

If no one has told you they loved you recently, tell that image **you love it BUT** you are going to become a new person so also tell that image **goodbye.**

Go to your kitchen, make a pot of coffee or tea if you prefer it, and fix yourself a decent breakfast, making sure to eat a good solid meal.

When you are through with your breakfast the real work begins.

Go outside, stretch expansively and take a deep breath of fresh air. Take that air as far down into your lungs as you can get it. Hold it down as long as you can do so, then release it slowly.

The first day the air may not go down really deeply without making you cough or hurt, but it will get easier as we go along. Then take another five or six deep breaths, stretch your muscles and start walking.

Oh, you haven't done that for some time, huh? It always left you short of breath and made the backs of your calves hurt?

All that was caused
by you smoking
too many cigarettes
for too many years.

Your circulation has decreased because of plaque buildup in your leg's arteries because you smoked and had bad dietary habits. This condition is known in the medical community as peripheral artery disease (PAD). But we are going to fix that aren't we?

While you are walking, stop every quarter mile or so—or more often if you need to—and take another series of deep breaths, holding them as long and as deeply as you can. Then exhale until all that stale air has been removed from your lungs. Keep deep breathing and exhaling until you have walked **half as far** as you think you can, because, remember, you also have to walk **BACK.** You might want to time yourself at first, 15 minutes out, 15 minutes back. If you can't walk far this first day, don't give up, just walk as far as you can, rest briefly, then return. But each day or so try to increase the distance you walk even if it is only a few steps or minutes farther. You will be amazed how soon you will be able to walk farther than you did the day before and with less effort. If for some reason you are unable to walk at all, as I was because of a physical disability, try going to a gym or YMCA and signing up for water aerobics classes. Attend each session and follow the instructor. But even in the water you should occasionally take the deep breathing exercises.

Due to my having damage in my legs from back surgery I preferred this method of exercise and really enjoyed it. The first two times I went my mobile oxygen tank and breathing apparatus went with me. On the third trip I didn't need it.

Within four months of water aerobics I got off the oxygen for at least 12 hours per day. Now I only use it at night.

I sincerely believe that my being on oxygen for terminal sleep apnea assisted me in not wanting to smoke again. Having that clean steady oxygen supply streaming into my lungs helped me to recover. If you feel that would help you and you can afford it or have insurance, talk with your doctor. You may not need it forever, but it does help you breathe better.

When you return from the gym or your walk, it is time for a shower. After that, eat a healthy lunch with a small portion of lean meat and some vegetables or a salad.

Is There Still More?

Yes, you betcha there is more. There's lots more. As soon as lunch is over and you have put your dishes into the dishwasher or cleaned them yourself, get cracking.

The first day you do not smoke we are going to fill a pail with plenty of warm soapy water. I would add some lemon scented cleanser to this if I were you. You will need all the help you can get.

We are going to start washing the walls of your living room since that is probably the place where you sit to smoke most of the time while you watch television.

First remove all the curtains and drapes from your windows. Drop your curtains in the washer and dryer while you clean the walls. Don't stop with the walls; wash and shine the windows and all the woodwork also. Why, you ask? Because if you are a smoker **your house stinks,** that is why.

Your house can be so clean you could eat off the proverbial commode or your floors as the old saying goes, but **it still stinks**. I know you will deny this to your dying day but I can assure you it does. You just can't smell it now, but one day in the not too distant future you will be able to I promise you that. Occasionally, look at your bucket of wash water. See how dirty it is, how greasy and almost sticky it appears? That is nicotine, tars and stale smoke pure and simple.

The inside of your lungs is filled with this same greasy stuff. That is why you cannot breathe well if you are a smoker and why you cough so much at the slightest exertion you make. You always tell people you are getting a cold, but in reality you have the old cigarette cough. One friend of mine, a heavy smoker, coughed so long and so hard his lung collapsed and he nearly died. That convinced him to stop smoking. Others have developed aortic aneurisms (a ballooning out of the largest artery in your body located below your heart).

After your walls, windows, woodwork and anything else not moving or biting you in your butt is clean, set up that ironing board and iron your curtains, then re-hang them. Dispose of the mini-blinds you took down because you will never get the smoke and nicotine off them. It is cheaper in the long run, if you really like the dust-catching things, to just replace them. I just threw my own away. They do look nice on your windows, but they catch every speck of cigarette smoke which sticks like glue to those little slats.

If you are still breathing after all this, stop and take several more deep breaths. You are going to need them because it is now time to vacuum and shampoo your carpet. While the carpet is drying you can wash, dry and then polish all your wood furniture, lamps and pictures in this room. Do you see where I am going with all this?

I know by now you are cussing me and calling me bad names but you needed to be pushed a little.

Every day we will clean another room because I assure you **every room** in your house **stinks**; even **your closets stink.** Even gifts wrapped in foil, stuffed inside a tightly sealed plastic bag, **stink!!** You may be the most finicky housekeeper on the block but I guarantee you if you smoke, your house stinks. So do the clothes inside your closets and even the sheets on your bed. We will launder them another day and sort and dispose of those items of clothing we no longer wear.

At supper time, if you are still standing erect, enjoy a normal meal but don't overdo it. You have had a lot of activity and exercise today so a relaxing meal will go over pretty well I expect.

If at any time during the day you feel a need for a cigarette, take a long drink of ice water instead. In fact, keep a glass handy and drink lots of it. Water is good for you and will help your body rid itself of the toxins smoking leaves in your bloodstream and we are routing from your body.

Add broccoli and cauliflower, bell peppers and lots of spinach and other green leafy vegetables to your daily diet. All these foods are delicious and assist in removing unwanted toxins from your blood. Eat some of these vegetables every day, either raw, slightly cooked or chopped in salads.

And, for goodness sakes, don't forget to take your vitamins. A multi-vitamin is a must. I also add extra calcium, and vitamins C, E, and B tablets every day.

I never felt I needed to take vitamins because I ate a good variety of foods that we grew in our garden, but once I started taking vitamins I could tell a world of difference after about 2 weeks.

If you are susceptible to colds, and I presume you are because of all the smoke going through your nasal passages and into your lungs, you might consider adding an echinacea tablet to your vitamin cocktail each day. Take this tablet for about two months, then take two months off, then repeat the dosage. It helps improve your immune system, but don't overdo it.

I read in a newspaper health column that echinacea shortened the duration of colds or prevented them entirely. I found this to be true. My husband, an outdoor worker and a former smoker of long standing, always had four or five severe colds each year. After adding echinacea to his vitamin cocktail each morning, he has not had a cold for several years. It was used by the Native Americans for hundreds of years to help them stay healthy.

Every day we are going to continue the exercise and cleaning routines. One of your concerns when you started was what you would do with your hands if you weren't smoking. Now you know what to do with them! Clean the nicotine off something in your home. Don't forget to take down the lamp covers from your ceiling light. A person I know had brown lamp covers. Once they were clear!!!!

Once the house is clean from floors to ceilings, clean your car. Empty and wash that overflowing ashtray. Yuck!! Clean upholstery and wash every inch of the inside with lemon freshener in your water. Then the outside can be washed, waxed and buffed.

Still need to find more to do? How about planting a new flower garden or weeding the old ones. Plant a flower bulb every time you want to light up a cigarette and watch your garden grow. This way you can watch your progress grow.

Or, if you smoked two packs every day, start a savings bank at home. Each day for one year that you do not smoke add into the bank the cost of those two packs. Never take any out. Watch your investment in yourself bloom. Now with the price of smokes being so expensive, you might now be able to afford a new car.

A recovering alcoholic I know has done this for years. Every time he wanted or needed a drink, he planted another bulb or plant. His flower gardens are now the showplace of the neighborhood.

During the Christmas season when he felt the urge to drink a cold one, he added another string of lights to his house, plants or trees in his yard. Now his place looks like the Griswold's house at Christmas time. Spruce up your yard. Plant, tend and harvest a vegetable garden. Those extra-fresh vegetables will come in handy in your new lifestyle and will save you a ton of money besides. The jobs are endless.

But whatever you do, **DO NOT** visit anyone who smokes, go where it is allowed, or allow a smoker to enter your home until after the first week is completed.

Paste a **"Do Not Smoke"** sign on your front door. Do not buy a pack of cigarettes and shove them **unopened** in a drawer.

Do not take that first puff.
Don't even pick up that
first unlit cigarette and twirl
it between two fingers.

Don't even handle a package of smokes. **You do not need them now.**

When you have gone a full week without smoking, congratulate yourself but keep up your exercise routine or continue at the gym and maintain the deep breathing exercises.

Now, don't you feel better already? I know you do. You just needed to be jump started. Tell that person in your mirror each morning that you are working on it.

After that first week is behind you, you literally have it made in the shade.

Treat yourself to a visit to your dentist for a dental cleaning.

Have your teeth cleaned and polished, maybe even whitened.

Did you ever think that your mouth tasted just like a stinking ashtray when someone kissed you? It did.

Cleaning your teeth and brushing your tongue and palate gently each time you brush your teeth will improve your kissability.

You are saving enough money by not buying cartons of cigarettes to easily pay for a visit to your dentist.

Go to your hairdresser and reward yourself with that new hair style you have been wanting. Using the money you have saved by not smoking you can spare the extra cash to get a new hair style.

I know your hair has been lank and stringy because it was so full of greasy nicotine you had to wash it every day and now it is as dry as straw.

What do you see now when you look in the mirror? Tell that person how swell he/she now looks.

I bet you can already see an improvement in your complexion. Are your eyes brighter? Friend, you are **over the hump** and you just lost 5 pounds this week with all that exercise. Your hands stayed busy too didn't they. Just remember to

NEVER TAKE THAT
FIRST PUFF
AFTER YOU QUIT

For the rest of your life you will be like a recovering alcoholic who cannot handle even one drink.

Take one puff
on a cigarette and
you will be hooked again.

I once quit for three years, picked up and smoked one cigarette from a friend's pack, and I was hooked again.

If you still feel you cannot do this alone, try asking a friend, smoking spouse or relative to go through the routine with you at the same time. This will give you someone to call if you feel yourself weakening and thinking about smoking.

Form a small support group, but do not run around telling everyone how you are quitting smoking. Let them find out for themselves when they see you sitting quietly, at rest, not needing a cigarette.

At the end of a year, treat yourself to a nice vacation on your banked savings.

I found that all the crutches devised by doctors and man to help me stop smoking were just that, crutches. Perhaps they will help you and if they do, go for it girl, but holding a sucker in my mouth all day made me look ridiculously childish and added to the weight gain. Everyone I met would say, "Oh, you are trying to quit smoking, eh?"

Trying was the operative word. I was "trying" but not succeeding. Cold turkey, exercise and love accomplished a miracle.

Good luck and God Bless.

Living Life by the Numbers

A No-Nonsense Approach to Managing Your Type II Diabetes

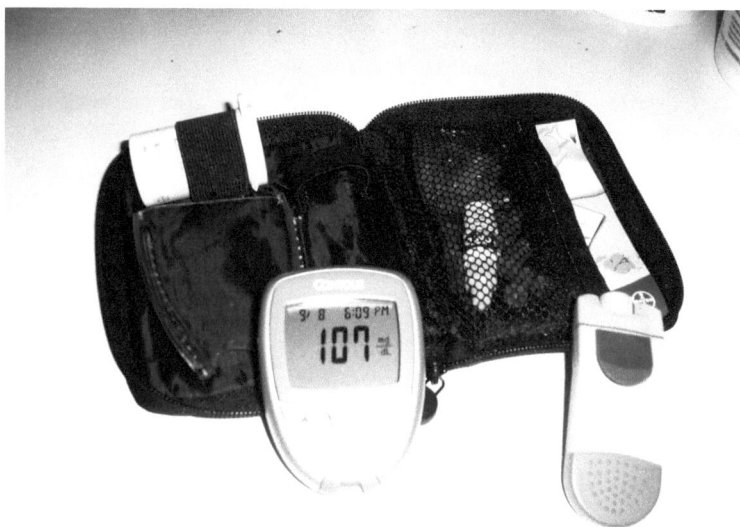

This booklet is neither sponsored nor endorsed by the American Diabetes Association.

It was written to illustrate to a friend what I have learned since being diagnosed with America's epidemic of Type II diabetes.

My Story

After being diagnosed with Type II diabetes, I tried for one year to follow my doctor's and the medical center dietitian's advice on how to control my disease. They recommended exercise and eating six to 11 servings of carbohydrates, three servings of protein and two servings of fats while eating three meals and one snack each day. What I learned from this quest was that eating this many carbohydrates every day made me gain more weight. And thus, my story begins.

After what I had thought would be a normal annual check-up visit with my doctor, the results were in; I, like so many millions of other Americans, was now a Type II diabetic. My lifestyle had to change and change quickly. For years I had wrestled with low blood sugar (hypoglycemia), but now I had switched over and become a full-fledged diabetic.

Not yet a grossly out-of-control diabetic—my high reading was only 126—I also had other risk factors. For years I had suffered with skin infections, abscesses, cracked dry feet, excessive thirst and fatigue, all of which are definitive descriptions of a true diabetic. My doctor suspected diabetes and ordered a complete blood count and took a urine sample. Her belief that I had diabetes was confirmed.

I returned from a visit with a dietitian armed with a small, hand-held instrument. It would tell me the amount of sugar (glucose) in my blood when a small drop of blood was placed on a plastic slide. I also was given a list of foods allowed from a food pyramid and the amounts needed to maintain a healthy blood glucose level. I was instructed to stick my finger and take a reading at least three or four times daily. My doctor also wrote me a prescription for a small pill called "Actos" which I was to take once every day. The pill was to assist me in the management of my disease.

Actos is only one of several prescription medications available for this disease. My doctor did not think I needed to be on insulin injections just yet.

Do not get upset if the first pill the doctor prescribes for you causes some unpleasant side effects or fails to control your diabetes. Discuss these problems with your doctor as soon as possible and ask to try another brand. It would be wise to request free samples until you find the one that works best for you with a minimal amount of side effects while still controlling your glucose level. Some of these medications are very expensive. No one pill works the same for every patient so some experimentation may be required.

You will need to work very closely with a caring physician after your diagnosis. This disease is not to be trifled with because it affects every system and organ in your body.

I had a friend, also recently diagnosed with Type II diabetes, who was totally confused, scared, depressed, embarrassed (diabetes was a "fat" disease, wasn't it?) and in the dark about what she should or should not eat, and the activities she could participate in. She did not have a clue as to how to recognize a carbohydrate. Typical questions you might have include, "Why do I have it? Did I "catch" it from someone? Did I inherit the disease? Had this writer passed the diabetes gene onto my two children, or my grandchildren?"

As I thought back on what diseases my parents and other friends had lived with I remembered my dad and a couple of my brothers had been diabetic. The brother of a friend had also suffered from renal (kidney) disease as a result of his diabetes; another friend had a lower limb amputated because of a circulatory problem related to diabetes. All had died fairly young, early 50's-70's age. The tendency to contract diabetes can be passed down from generation to generation or it may skip one generation and hit the next.

If both parents had the disease, then a child is doubly cursed with the propensity to have diabetes and must take evasive actions over their entire life span to try to prevent it.

The more I learned about diabetes, the healthier I became.

I learned that there are two kinds of diabetes. Type I is normally detected in childhood and happens when the pancreas (which produces insulin) fails to do its job. This is commonly called childhood diabetes and it is very dangerous. Type I may also occur later in life, but that is rarer.

Type II is usually detected later in life, but more and more often Type II diabetes is being detected in our overweight young children. The pancreas may still be working, but the cells in the body have trouble utilizing the insulin. They are said to be "insulin resistant" and must be assisted by exercise, diet and medication.

Insulin is the enzyme your body utilizes to carry energy produced by the food you eat to all the cells of your body. But sometimes the cells do not accept this energy and thus the energy, think of calories, is deposited elsewhere as fat in the body— thereby compounding the problem. A good analogy of this process might be a mother feeding her child. She might sit the child in a high chair and with a spoon (the insulin) bring the food to the baby's mouth. The child (the cell in this case) turns its head and compresses its lips, denying itself what it needs to live. The mother then places the food from the spoon onto a plate and leaves it there and tries again. The cell (child) eventually dies from starvation yet there are mounds of food everywhere for it to eat.

The most commonly accused culprits for causing diabetes is a sedentary (lazy) lifestyle and too much food. More and more Americans are eating away from home each day contrary to the way they ate in earlier generations.

The diet of the early humans was limited primarily to the foods they grew, hunted, produced and preserved. It was cooked and eaten in their caves and in later years in their homes. These earlier foods contained a lot of fiber, often very dense complex carbohydrates and fatty meats. These people generally were much more active than we are today and needed this excess caloric intake to survive. It took enormous amounts of energy just to get through every day but they burned far greater amounts of calories than today's people do. Yet most of us still eat these enormous amounts of calories which we no longer need for survival.

As our industrial revolution continued, we found more and more ways to process, crush, roll and refine our foods to an even finer texture until nothing was left but the sugars at the core of the grain. We eventually processed the fiber and bran right out of most of our foods and it tasted great. Those pies, cakes and cookies and other baked products made from processed white flour taste so good that it is a rare person who can resist eating them. Now, instead of being hunters and gatherers, we are eating food with less and less fiber and substance, thus the rise in diabetes. Prior to this time when a family needed flour or cornmeal the father would place sacks of corn or wheat that he had grown and harvested himself into a wagon and take it to a grist mill to be turned into meal and flour. These mills used huge round grinding stones which generally were powered by water running across a water wheel but the flour and meal thus produced contained all the nutrients of the whole grain that are lacking in today's foods. I believe the big problems arose during and just after the Second World War.

During that time period, thousands of women who had been homemakers their entire lives went to work in factories, turning out war material. They were now earning a nice paycheck and many of them enjoyed having the freedom and control of their own money which in the past had been relegated to the males of her household.

But by leaving her home to work she had less and less time to spend at home tending and feeding her family. So what did she do? She no longer raised a garden to feed her family but shopped at grocery stores to supply her pantry.

The nation's food processing plants answered her call for more and more products that she could take down from a shelf and cook for her family. But to make that food last longer once it was canned, and to allow it to retain its color and texture, many things were added and taken away from that food. Food preservatives and colors were added as were fats, salt and sugars. The food looked like it should in its natural state and most had some nutritional value, but the danger lay in not knowing all the hidden ingredients. In the past when she had preserved her own garden produce and butchered her own meats the housewife knew exactly what was in a can of her food that was opened. Now she no longer had that knowledge.

Today's rules about labeling answer many of the questions we might have, but the labeling needs updating as we become smarter.

Then along came the nation's saturation of fast food chains on nearly every street corner and bingo, the scourge was on. Instead of walking to the fields and working hard all day, people could now rise from their beds later in the morning, and rush to work in their air conditioned or warm vehicles. They could pull into a fast food drive-thru and order bacon, egg and cheese biscuits with hash brown potatoes, maybe two orders if they were really hungry and a cup of café au lait.

Once at their desk they loaded down with several more cups of coffee and probably smoked several cigarettes. This got them through until their break or noon hour when they would discover they were hungry again. They might even eat a bag of chips or a package of cookies or snack crackers during break to hold them until lunch.

Going through the drive-thru at a different chain for lunch, they ordered three pieces of fried and breaded chicken, mashed potatoes and gravy, another biscuit, perhaps even an order of baked beans or pasta and a 44 ounce glass of soda sweetened with sugar or a milkshake. Taking this back to their workplace, it was consumed.

By 3 p.m. they were exhausted and could hardly keep their eyes open. Their carbohydrates had "kicked in" and no wonder! In other words, their blood glucose level had spiked and had by then fallen to the bottom of the scale. It was difficult to concentrate and they were very tired and sleepy.

At quitting time they rushed home to a sit down or take-out supper with their spouse and kids so all could hurry to the television set or computer and sit until bedtime. But before bedtime, they found they must make one final raid on the refrigerator. Maybe there was a piece of pie or a chicken leg remaining and there was no use letting it go to waste; it would ruin and turn stale by the next day. So that would be eaten also and it would still go to waist.

Now there is a glut of restaurant buffets in which you can stretch your gut at almost any hour of the day. For about $7 per person you can eat until you are ready to pop. There will be six to ten kinds of meats served along with a couple dozen vegetables, soups, breads, tons of salads, berries, melons and of course, don't forget the dessert and ice cream bar. How can a cook compete with this variety for her family at this low cost? Everyone can eat what they want and they are happy.

It is no wonder that so many of our people are fat. I have seen pre-teen children go around these buffet lines with their plate taking servings from the bars four and five times. They might drink half a dozen glasses of full-sugared sodas to wash it down and then go to the dessert bar and load up there.

In earlier times dining out was reserved for very special occasions such as family anniversaries or holidays. People would wear their best bib and tucker and go to a sit-down restaurant where they would be seated by an attendant and served individual portions of food. Desserts were available for additional fees.

When a child comes home from school or a parent comes home from work today they quickly eat from either carry out or boxed and partially prepared foods in front of their television set or computers. The parents will be watching silly sitcoms and the child may be in his own room playing video games on his many electronic toys or watching television there.

Both adults and children believe it is too hot/ too cold/ etc. to be outside so they sit in their climate controlled homes all the time. Their homes are centrally heated and cooled with furnaces that require no assistance. The family members no longer have even the evening chore of carrying in wood/coal or loading it into the furnace to do. With the mere twist of a dial or finger on a keypad we can just dial up the amount of heat or cold air we want inside our homes.

Many of the children of today do not actually know how to play outside anymore.

My sister tells the story about two of her grandsons who lived next door to her and spent time at her house when they were youngsters. Rather than let them sit in front of the television set or play video games for hours on end, she said she would make them go outside for 30 minutes to expend their energy and get some fresh air as she had had to do as a youngster herself.

She said she overheard one say to the other one day, "I wonder what we are supposed to do out here?" With their hands in their pockets they stood outside until, banging on her door to get her attention and ask if they could come back inside, she told them they could. Isn't that a sad story? They did not know what to do outdoors for play.

They had never chased and caught lightening bugs and placed them in a jar to watch them blink on and off or played lawn croquet or climbed trees. They didn't have a clue how to play hide and seek, Annie Over, tag or many of the other games popular when we were young that burned off our excess calories.

Does any of this sound familiar? It happens millions of times every day.

What can you do? How can you avoid getting diabetes in the first place? Or, once you have it, how do you manage it? How do you play the numbers game?

First things first. The first thing you do of course, is ask questions to find out what diabetes is. Your doctor, nurse practitioner or a friend who already has the disease can help you understand a great deal.

What Is
a Carbohydrate?

You must learn what a carbohydrate is. Many people have no idea exactly what a carbohydrate is when you ask them about it. A friend told this writer that she believed a carbohydrate was anything white, thinking only of potatoes, rice and white bread. So she had changed to eating whole-wheat toast for breakfast. When buying bread one should look for a label that says 100 percent whole grain, not just whole wheat as the product's first ingredient; stone-ground whole grain is even better. Our food labeling regulations state that the ingredients must be listed in their order of prominence with the one used most in that product listed first. So my friend was right to an extent, she just didn't carry it out far enough.

A lot of people have asked me, "What is a carbohydrate?" I do my best to educate and let others know what little I have learned. My knowledge has been hard won. I have studied information about my disease in books, on the Internet, from other friends, my doctor and others. All of this research takes time. If someone who already knows the answers can put it in an easily understandable language, it greatly simplifies things and you can be up and running very quickly. To make it simple, a carbohydrate is any food that contains sugar, gluten or starch. All three are easily, quickly and readily digested and turned into sugar once eaten. Such foods as corn, beans, white bread, peas, potatoes, rice and some other cereals, pasta and more are starches, thus they are also carbohydrates. They can be of several colors other than white, but they are still a starch, therefore a sugar. A starch turns into sugar soon after it is consumed. But there are a lot of good carbohydrates (complex) and then there are bad carbohydrates (simple).

All carbohydrates are not bad for you. They are required by your brain, muscles and other organs as an energy source. Without carbohydrates you could not survive. But an excess of bad carbohydrate leads to fat being stored in your body's cells, leading eventually to diabetes and other related "fat diseases."

A serving of carbohydrates has been determined to equal 15 grams. You have to read every label in your pantry to discover the food that contains the amount of carbohydrates you may consume. For example, one slice of white bread is one serving of carbohydrate. Until you can easily determine how much a ½ cup serving is, (a 1/2 cup serving equals one serving of carbohydrate) measure the food. After a while you can pretty well guess how much constitutes one serving of any food.

Proteins and fats are other types of foods required for good health and are digested and handled differently by your body. This food group contains meat and eggs, milk, cheese, nuts and other foods. There are nine grams in one serving of protein and a serving is equal in size to a deck of cards or the palm of your hand. They take much longer to digest; thus eating more protein and cutting back on carbohydrates will prevent your body's blood glucose level from spiking.

Another food group includes melons, fruits and berries. While these need to be included in a healthy diet, some are high in sugar except for the berries. Blueberries, strawberries and raspberries are excellent for any diet. They can be eaten as desserts or added to salads or cereals very easily. Melons are slightly higher in calories, but excellent choices over sugar-laden sweets because they contain a lot of beta carotene. If you like fruit, eat the actual fruit because that way you consume more fiber. Consumed as juices they are highly concentrated sugars with much of the fiber removed and so should be used judiciously.

Dr. Atkin's New Diet Revolution book was a godsend for me. The day I completed reading the Atkins book I had also taken my diabetes medicine that morning. About 2 p.m. I realized my vision had blurred and I was becoming jittery.

I remembered that the diet book said the blood glucose level must be monitored closely when starting this high protein, low carb type of diet. I arrayed the equipment and checked my glucose level; it read 49. I had eaten few if any carbs that day according to Dr. Atkin's instructions and had taken my medication. The combination had lowered my glucose level far too low.

A "normal" blood glucose reading is anything from 80-120. These numbers may be lowered soon, I recently read. Remembering what Dr. Atkins had written, I quickly got a very small amount of protein and ate it. About 15 minutes later I felt much better and my new reading was 79. After testing and tracking my "numbers" for about 3 months, I no longer had to check my blood every day, and I had been off medication from day two; and in the first 28 days had lost a total of 17 pounds.

This pamphlet is not an endorsement of any particular diet or diet book. It just happens that this writer had just completed reading Dr. Atkin's New Diet Revolution book at the urging of her son who loved to investigate foods and their effects on the human body. However, it did work for me. There is no such thing as a diet, rather there are different ways in which to enjoy food. Two full years after cutting back on carbohydrates, my blood sugar level remains between 80-100 and I no longer have to monitor more than three or four times per month. My doctor cut my required visits from every three months to every six months.

There are several good books on the market which can help with diabetes control. Buy them and read them; digest what they are telling you. It is imperative that you learn to read food labels and it is fun to experiment with a lot of different new foods. You may find a new food you love. Next on my list of foods to try is grilled eggplant. If you need more help in reading food labels, don't hesitate to call your local County Extension Office. They may have a class you can attend or if they are not too busy, they may sit down with you and explain how to read the labels. I have found our Extension Agent to be very knowledgeable and helpful.

There is an excellent book containing the glycemic index of different foods on the market. Be sure to read one and you will better understand which carbohydrates cause your blood sugars to spike. Try to keep a pocket sized carbohydrate book in your purse to reference when you are dining out. The one this writer uses also gives the nutritional values of several menu items when eating at fast food restaurants. You may eat out occasionally, but do so cautiously.

Learn to choose and prepare foods in a more healthy way. For instance, substituting olive or canola oil for lard will make a tremendous difference in the way you feel and how food tastes. Make your own salad dressing or get brave and not use any; instead add berries or a chopped apple and a bit of lemon juice or a spice called Accent in place of dressing.

Most of those little packages of dressing provided in restaurants and the bottles on our grocer's shelves are killers to anyone's diet. Read the labels on the back of the package. They are loaded with fats, oils and sugars and can turn what was once a healthy salad into a dangerous food. The buttermilk ranch is one of the lesser destructive dressings. Some of the sweeter red ones contain about 400 calories per packet and tons of fat and I have seen some people pour two or three packets or more on a chef's salad.

Instead of making plain macaroni and cheese, I add lots of broccoli and a few chopped carrots to cut down on the carbs to make the dish more diabetic friendly. There are many tricks like this you can learn and use.

You can bake or broil meats instead of frying. Or try stir frying thin strips of chicken or lean beef with lots and lots of fresh vegetables and mushrooms. This is also delicious using only the roasted vegetables. I also purchased an air fryer. It does not need any oil and takes less than 10 minutes to make fresh French fries. This is a low-fat alternative way of cooking that is absolutely delicious. Invest now in a wok or a large very deep non-stick skillet.

Stir-frying and non-stick skillets and pans require only a minimal amount of oil. Leave off ladling the stir fry over a bed of rice or noodles. Do not add any of the commercially prepared Oriental dressings to your stir fry. They are loaded with oil, salt and sugars. Just eat a big bowl or even two of these vegetables with the little bites of meat and maybe a handful of roasted nuts for a satisfying meal containing very few calories. Never overcook your vegetables; leave them a bit crisp; chewing burns calories and leaves you feeling full longer!

Instead of soft drinks which are loaded with either sugar or sugar substitutes, try some of the packaged soft drink mixes. Wyler's, Crystal Lite and Wal-Mart's Great Value brand among others has several nice fruit and tea flavors from which to choose. These drinks contain sugar substitutes but they lack the carbonated fizz of sodas. Try the different store brands and flavors, which are sometimes less expensive, until you discover which ones you prefer and use those instead of soda.

Better yet, just drink more water. It has no caffeine, and no calories or other unhealthy ingredients and will be much better for you than diet soda. Sugar substitutes may cause some unpleasant reactions in some people who drink many diet sodas every day. You might even try some of the flavored sparkly water for a nice change. Whether or not you are watching your diet you need to drink at least 64 ounces of water a day to remove excess debris and toxins from your system.

Cut back on caffeine consumption and stop smoking. Change your lifestyle and become more active. Due to having crippled knees from botched back surgery, and then having a blood clot in my left groin, this writer found that attending water aerobics class was the answer. If your community has no public pool like a YMCA or park, check with the local motels and schools to see if they have a pool privilege package they will sell you. Some motels will even let you use their pool free if you use it very early in the morning before their guests arise. Just get active in the water even if they have no instructor. You will be totally amazed how much better you feel.

For those who can afford it, or live in an area where there is no public pool, try installing an endless pool in a small area of your home's basement or in an outbuilding so you can exercise in the water every day. The pools can be fitted into most basements and cost about $20,000 I believe according to literature I have seen. If you have one piece of home exercise equipment and you have friends who have others, form a club. Each day you exercise, go to a different home and work out on a different machine. You may have to run a classified ad in your local newspaper or ask friends to find someone who will work out with you.

Will doing all the above things cure your diabetes? No, it will not, but switching to even one or two new practices will help you deal with your disease and help you lower your "numbers." Trying these things may also help you prevent the disease if you have not yet been diagnosed with diabetes. But once you have been diagnosed, if you follow your doctor's advice, take your medications as directed (the dosages may have to be lowered if you follow this high protein/low carb food advice) and lose weight (even losing a few pounds will make a difference) you should be able to live a fuller, healthier life.

Keep a diary of your glucose readings and the food you eat if necessary. If you eat a big holiday meal, for instance, make a notation in the diary. Wait 30 minutes after eating, test and write down your numbers. Learn which foods cause your glucose level to spike and which ones have little or no effect on your numbers and eat more of those kinds.

This writer learned that eating an ice cream cone occasionally had no effect on her readings the day she ate it but made her fatigued the next day. A slice of pie or cake or cookies or candy sent the spike on its merry way upwards very quickly. Eating sugar is not the cause of diabetes we are told but giving sweets to a diabetic is like offering a recovering alcoholic a drink.

I also have learned to substitute stone-ground whole wheat flour and cornmeal in my baking instead of white processed flour and meal. The stone-ground products do not make your numbers spike because they are a very highly complex form of grain and have a very nice, nutty taste.

It is up to YOU to take charge of your health. If you remember nothing else I have said in this booklet, remember that last sentence.

Your doctor is a busy person. He or she may not always remember what you are allergic to or even what is wrong with you. They can and do make mistakes. They have a lot of patients. You have only one patient to worry about, YOURSELF. If you think of a question to ask your doctor between visits, write it down and take it with you on your next visit. No question is dumb. It is only dumb if you neglect to ask it. Or better yet, if you feel an answer to your question is vitally important, call and speak with the office nurse, explain your question concisely, and ask the doctor to respond as soon as possible.

You should not be a hypochondriac and call the doctor every day, because they may then begin to avoid you. Experience says that a clearly worded query to the doctor will get results. They seem to appreciate it when you ask questions and report clearly the nature of your symptoms.

Also, remember to keep an eye on the health of your feet. They are the first extremity to go bad when you are diabetic. Check your feet every day. If necessary see a podiatrist on a regular basis. Medicare pays for foot care for the older diabetic. You might want to check and see if they will also pay for you. Some friends and I have learned it is both fun and less expensive to have a pedicure than see the doctor for toenail trimming, oiling and softening of the feet.

Also, see your eye doctor at least once each year and your dentist twice a year. Advise both of them you are a diabetic. A diabetic will sometimes have hemorrhages in the back of the eyeball. Remember that diabetes is the leading cause of blindness in adults. Doctors are learning that tooth problems may be indicative of heart problems, so see that dentist and keep flossing. Know what your normal urine output is and record any changes to report to your doctor. Producing very little, or very dark urine, is an emergency and should be reported to your doctor immediately. You may have gone into renal insufficiency. This is a life-threatening condition.

Some doctors recommend you keep a packet of candy, crackers, glucose tubes or other food in your purse, office or car in case you feel jittery which means your glucose has dropped too low.

I have found through trial and error on this quest for knowledge about diabetes that a protein bar works better for me. You will have to experiment with this idea. If I am going to be somewhere and miss a meal, I will use a meal replacement bar with a bottle of cold water or a protein "milkshake" to take the place of a meal. There are many of these products on the market and several are very tasty and satisfying.

Try to find single nutrition bars to taste test before you buy any particular brand in quantity. Several small meals on a regular schedule are far better than three large meals daily. Some dieticians recommend no more than 5 hours between meals to regulate the needs of diabetics. Diabetes plays a number on every system and organ in the body. It is an insidious disease with far reaching problems. You must be monitored closely, and the best monitor of your body is YOU. If you are having problems and your doctor is not available, go to an emergency room at once.

I ask that you show a copy of this booklet to your health care provider. I have tried to be honest and straight forward in sharing what I have learned. If they disagree with anything I have presented, please ask them to contact me at the telephone number at the bottom of this paper. It was written to help a friend who has the disease much worse than I do to get started. I have been researching this disease and reading about it for nearly three years. I do not claim to be an expert on the disease, but feel I am now an expert on MY body.

To help you get started on a different lower carb way to eat, there are some recipes that I have developed attached to this pamphlet. All are delicious and even your family will probably want to share the results, so prepare plenty!

Preparing Your Food

To prepare yourself for a new way of eating will require a trip to the produce and lean meat sections of your favorite grocery store. Give yourself plenty of time to look over and evaluate your possible selections.

We have eaten "fresh" for several years now and have found that we now buy very few canned food products except for juices and chili makings. We buy only the leanest cuts of meat. You may have to shop more often in order to keep up your supply of the fresh things because most refrigerator produce bins are kind of skimpy when you add a quantity of bulky items. Try to shop stores that are running produce and lean meat sales and stock up then to cut down on expenses.

Broccoli, cauliflower and bell peppers may be purchased in bulk and frozen for the soup and stir-fry featured below. All you have to do is wash, chop, blanch (except the peppers, they do not need to be blanched) cool and bag before freezing. To save even more time I bag enough of each of these items together in one large bag to make a batch of soup or stir-fry. I prefer it not having been frozen when I use these vegetables in salads.

These recipes may be shared if you find them helpful. Good eating and enjoy your life.

Recipe Section

Taco Salad. Chop about 2 or 3 cups of lettuce (I prefer to use romaine lettuce since its shelf life is longer and it is more crisp than head lettuce) and arrange in center of a plate. Around the edges place a few green olives and several grapes or chopped slicing tomatoes. Cover the lettuce with 1/3 cup shredded cheese. In a small pan, heat one can of chili w/no beans until heated through and pour over the cheese. Add several dots of Tabasco sauce and a dollop of sour cream. Do not use chips or crackers. This makes a huge meal. I don't eat a lot of beef, but you can brown and drain about 1/4 pound of ground beef and add it to the sauce if you like. Serves 1.

Fresh Spinach With Onion & Garlic. This sounds gross and smells bad while it is cooking but I assure you it is delicious. In a medium sized pan add 3 tablespoons of olive oil; 1 chopped medium onion and 2 cloves of minced garlic. Cook until the onion becomes opaque. Add coarse salt to taste and a 1 pound bag of frozen spinach. Cover and cook slowly until the spinach is heated through stirring now and then. If more moisture is needed, I add 1/3 cup white wine. I prefer to use frozen spinach for this recipe because the fresh kind reduces down to about one-half cup. The frozen variety gives you a full pound of greens.

Breakfast Quichlet. Spray a 9 x 13-inch baking dish with non-stick cooking spray. Add enough raw broccoli florets to cover the bottom to about a ½ inch depth. In a skillet brown 1 pound of lean sausage, drain well, and sprinkle over the broccoli. Sauté 1 ½ cups each chopped onion, chopped red and green bell peppers and sliced mushrooms in a teaspoon of olive oil. Sauté until onions are slightly clear. Sprinkle over the sausage. In a large bowl place 8 eggs, salt and pepper to taste, and a bit of heavy cream and beat until fluffy. Pour over the ingredients in the pan. Bake in a preheated 350-degree oven until the center is set (about 45 minutes). During the last 15 minutes cooking time, sprinkle top with shredded cheddar cheese. To serve, place each portion on a lettuce leaf on a plate, dot with Tabasco sauce and a dollop of sour cream. Add 5 or 6 olives to the plate and a couple slices of tomatoes. Makes 8-10 servings. This recipe is high in protein and fats, but I believe it corresponds with Dr. Atkin's diet guidelines. It is handy to prepare ahead of time (except for the eggs) if you are expecting guests and want to save time by preparing it the night before. I put the eggs on the morning I intend to serve it.

Beef Vegetable Soup. Cut a lean round steak that is about ½

inch thick into bite size pieces and place in a large pot containing 2 quarts of water and one 15 ounce can tomato sauce. Add one large chopped onion and 1 cup each chopped bell pepper and dried sliced mushrooms; 2 large carrots chopped; 2 tablespoons chopped chives; 1 tablespoon parsley flakes; and salt and pepper to taste. Cook until the meat is nearly fork tender. Add 3 cups each broccoli florets, cauliflower florets and diced cabbage. Cook until tender but leave the vegetables a bit crisp for better flavor. This recipe will make a lot of soup. You may divide it into individual servings and freeze it but at our house everyone loves it so well there is seldom any left over to freeze. It is high in vegetable content and very low in fat. Watch how much salt you use because these vegetables do not require much salt.

Boca Burger Swiss Steak. Brown a couple of Boca Burgers in a teaspoon of oil. Add these vegetable burgers to your favorite swiss steak or beef stew recipe (See recipe below). **NOTE**: Boca burgers are a soy meat substitute with the texture and taste of real meat and are found in the frozen meat aisle of your grocery.

Regular Swiss Steak. Cut a large round steak that is about ½ inch thick into 4 ounce pieces. Marinate overnight in teriyaki sauce. Roll the steak lightly in flour and brown quickly in hot oil, then place the pieces into a medium sized pot. Add one 15-ounce can tomato sauce; 2 cups water; 2 tablespoons chives; 1 tablespoon parsley flakes; 1 tablespoon diced garlic; 1 cup sliced mushrooms; and salt and pepper to taste. Cook until the steak is fork tender and the sauce has thickened. If it doesn't thicken enough, mix 2-tsp. cornstarch in a small amount of cold water and add this to the boiling sauce while stirring constantly. You may substitute 2 tablespoons of barley instead of the cornstarch mixture if you desire. This sauce makes excellent gravy to pour over mashed or baked potatoes for those in your household who can still enjoy potatoes.

Chef's Salad. Cut up as much of each ingredient from the following list as you like for your salad. I use all the following in proportions we have decided we enjoy. Lettuce, as many types as you want; broccoli and cauliflower florets; baby carrots in strips, onions; radishes; colored bell peppers, (two or three colors is best); grape tomatoes; white mushrooms; celery; radicchio (a red and white lettuce with a tangy flavor); sliced boiled eggs; pepperoni; soynuts; sunflower seeds; shredded cheddar cheese; and raisins. If you have another salad vegetable you enjoy add it, if you don't like one of these, omit it. Use a lemon juice and oil dressing (see next recipe). The soynuts take the place of croutons and add some crackle and protein to the salad.

Lemon Juice and Olive Oil Dressing. In a cruet place 1 packet of artificial sweetener; ½ teaspoon each salt, black pepper, chipped dried chives and garlic powder; 3 tablespoons water and 1/4 cup lemon juice (may use lemon concentrate). Shake to mix well. Fill cruet within 1 inch of top with olive oil and shake vigorously until all is mixed. Use sparingly because of the oil. Or get creative. Add a chopped apple or some ripe berries to the salad greens and forget the dressing.

Sautéed Cabbage. Preheat a large non-stick pan or skillet to medium and add a small dollop of butter. Chop a half head of cabbage into small pieces; add one medium, chopped, cored but unpeeled apple. Add cabbage and apple and a bit of salt and pepper to butter and cover; cook very slowly until crisp tender, stirring occasionally. I can smell it now. Scrumptious.

I have written a tried and true recipe book you might like to order from Amazon. "Grandma's Brown County Cookbook." Current selling price will be listed on Amazon.com. This cookbook contains scores of recipes including several for low carb dieters and tons of funny stories and lots of pretty pictures.

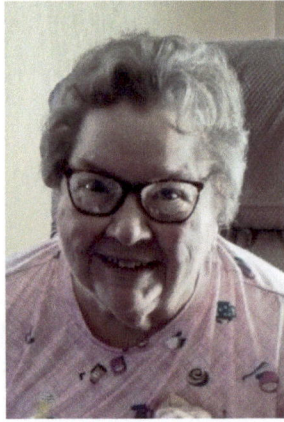

About the Author

Mrs. Ayers, a retired award- winning journalist, recently wrote and published two historical non-fiction books. A final historical book is now available titled, "This is Our Brown County." She retired from newspaper management in 1993 due to health problems explained in this booklet. A former Emergency Medical Technician she feels qualified to write about excesses in the medical field.

Extra copies of this book may be obtained by mailing $20 to cover the cost of printing and mailing to: **Health,**

7256 Keith Donaldson Road, Freetown, IN 47235. Please allow two weeks for delivery.

My E-Mail address is: hayers7256@yahoo.com.

About the Book

This is a hard-hitting exposé of our health care industry. It explores the problems encountered by the author when her doctor's inappropriate care nearly claimed her life. It is written as a warning to others and to spur the medical industry to higher standards. If you are contemplating becoming a hospital patient in the near future, **reading this book may save your life.**

The second part of the book should be read by everyone wanting to kick the nicotine habit. When you or a loved one succeed in breaking the nicotine habit after reading this booklet, and you can if my advice is followed, please drop me a letter or postcard and tell me about your experience. I would love to know I have helped you kick this nasty habit.

The third portion of this book explains how the author was able to tame her Type II diabetes by following a high protein, lower carbohydrate diet. It also provides some tasty recipes.

www.ingramcontent.com/pod-product-compliance
Lightning Source LLC
Chambersburg PA
CBHW040127270326
41927CB00001B/10